Model Mommy

EMMAUS PUBLIC LIBRARY
11 EAST MAIN STREET
EMMAUS, PA 18049

Model Mommy

Vendela's Plan for Emotional Support, Exercise,
and Eating Right After Having a Baby

To Emmaus Public Library, all the best

VENDELA

Vendela

Contemporary Books

Chicago New York San Francisco Lisbon London Madrid Mexico City
Milan New Delhi San Juan Seoul Singapore Sydney Toronto

Library of Congress Cataloging-in-Publication Data

Vendela.
    Model mommy : Vendela's plan for emotional support, exercise, and eating right after having a baby / Vendela.
       p.   cm.
    Includes index.
    ISBN 0-07-138484-7
      1. Motherhood.   2. Postnatal care.   3. Exercise for women.
    4. Physical fitness for women.   I. Title.

RG801.V46   2002
618.6—dc21   2002020793

Contemporary Books
A Division of The McGraw·Hill Companies

Copyright © 2002 by Sunflower Sun, Inc. All rights reserved. Printed in the United States of America. Except as permitted under the United States Copyright Act of 1976, no part of this publication may be reproduced or distributed in any form or by any means, or stored in a database or retrieval system, without the prior written permission of the publisher.

1 2 3 4 5 6 7 8 9 0   KGP/KGP   1 0 9 8 7 6 5 4 3 2

ISBN 0-07-138484-7

This book was set in Sabon
Printed and bound by Quebecor Kingsport
Cover and interior design by Nick Panos
Cover photo copyright © Anders Haggstrom
Hair: Jan Thomas for La Bionda
Stylist: Inge Marie Amedal
Makeup: Hilde Berntsen
Interior illustrations by Susy Pilgrim Waters
Interior photos: Pages x and xiv copyright © Andrew Eccles
Pages xii, xvii, xviii, xxi, xxii, xxiii, and 27 copyright © Adam Roberts
Page xv copyright © Curto Paolo/Sports Illustrated
Pages xix and 32 copyright © UNICEF
Page 11 copyright © Patrick Demarchelier, Inc.
Pages 13 and 14 copyright © Mona Nordoy
Pages 38, 46–55, 64–88, 92, 93, 94, 95 copyright © Jean Renard
All other photos copyright © Anders Haggstrom

McGraw-Hill books are available at special quantity discounts to use as premiums and sales promotions, or for use in corporate training programs. For more information, please write to the Director of Special Sales, Professional Publishing, McGraw-Hill, Two Penn Plaza, New York, NY 10121-2298. Or contact your local bookstore.

This book is printed on acid-free paper.

*This book is dedicated to the three people in the world
who mean the most to me: Julia, Hannah, and Olaf.
You give me sunshine even when it rains.*

Contents

Acknowledgments ix
Introduction xi

PART ONE Emotional Rescue

1. Hello Hormones, Good-Bye Serenity! 3
2. The Hardest Job You'll Ever Love 9
3. A Marriage of Minds 17
4. Boosting Your Body Image 25
5. If You Decide to Breast-Feed 31

PART TWO Exercise for Life

6. Find Your Motivation 39
7. Choose an Activity You Like 43
8. Time to Get Moving! Begin with Stretching 47
9. Cardio Work 57
10. Strength Training 65
11. Exercising with Your Baby 89

PART THREE Eating for One Again

12. Enjoying Your Food 99
13. Keep Healthy Food—and Only Healthy Food—on Hand! 103
14. Indulge Yourself! 109

PART FOUR Cooking for the Whole Family

15. Cooking for Two and a Half 117
16. My Favorite Healthy Recipes 123
17. Cooking Your Own Baby Food 151

Appendix 153
Index 159

Acknowledgments

This book would not have been possible without the help of my family and friends. First, thanks to my family: Olaf, Julia, and Hannah. Also Mamma, Pappa, and Tante Ingrid.

Thanks for help and contributions go to Rebecca Ascher-Walsh, Sean Kelleher, Katherine Petrillo, Sarah Hall, Cathy Quinn, Colby Hewitt, Elizabeth Lahey, Janet Crown-Peterson, Anders Haggstrom, Linda Hagen at Dugg, Jean Renard, Andrew Eccles, Leeann Patterson, Mona Nordoy, Patrick Demarchelier, Adam Roberts, Jan Mun, Jan Thomas, Inge Marie Amedal, Camilla Lökholm, Kristin Arnesen, Hilde Berntsen, Mary Cahill, and my friends at UNICEF. Also my gratitude to Thale Treider-Bonesmo for inspiration and to my editor, Judith McCarthy, for believing in this book and giving it a home.

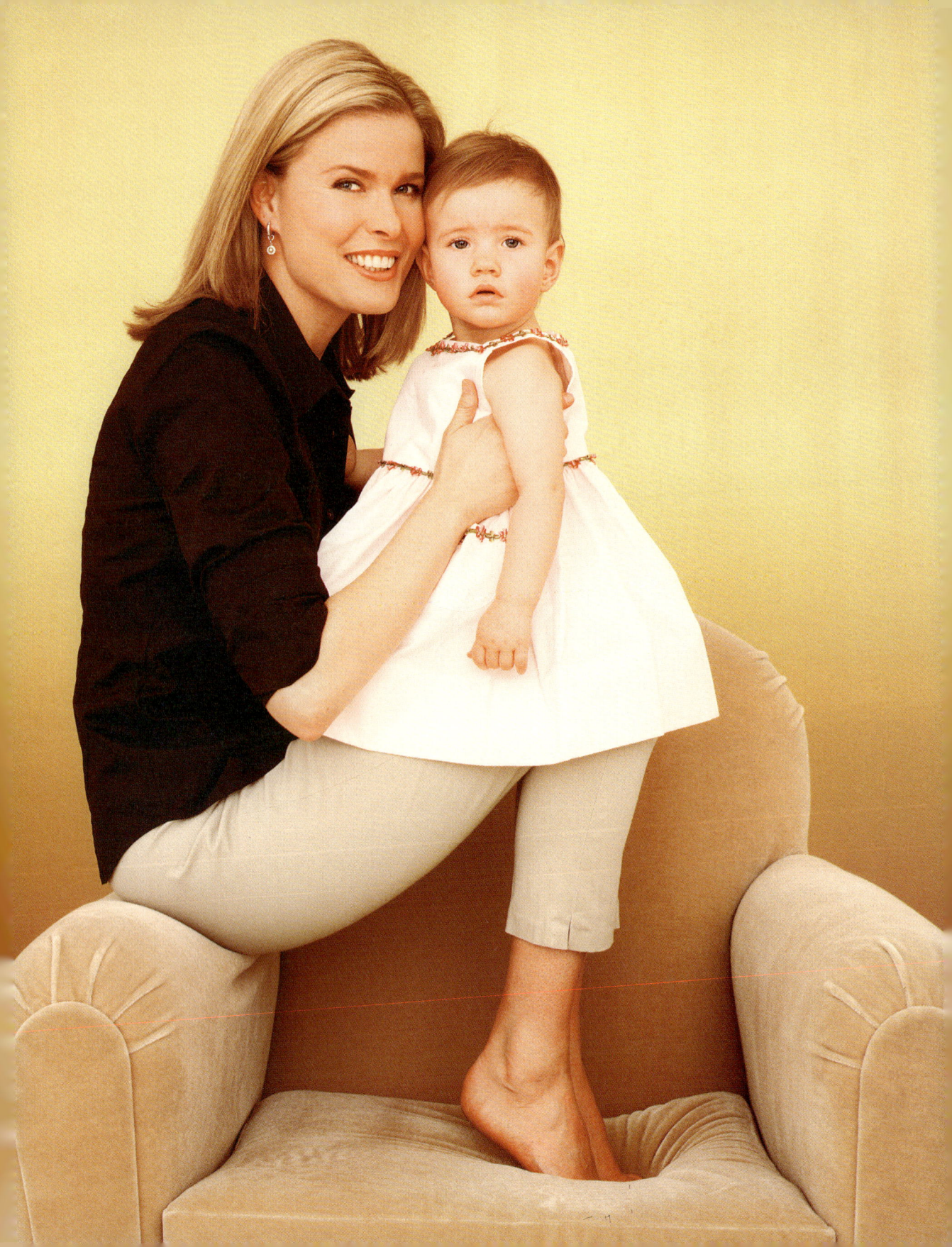

Introduction

Congratulations—you're a mother! Welcome to the adventure of a lifetime, an adventure you've imagined, dreamed about, and looked forward to for at least nine months.

What's amazing is that while you've probably never anticipated or planned for anything as much as you have the arrival of your new baby, so few of your fantasies come close to preparing you for the *hugeness* (no pun intended) of being a new mom.

Over the next few months, you will have days when you've never been happier, never felt more alive, never experienced such a deep love as you do for your child. Now that he's also the father of your child, you'll feel a stronger bond with your husband than you ever have before. You'll have a deeper respect for your body than you ever thought possible, because it carried this beautiful child to term. But then, you're probably counting on these feelings.

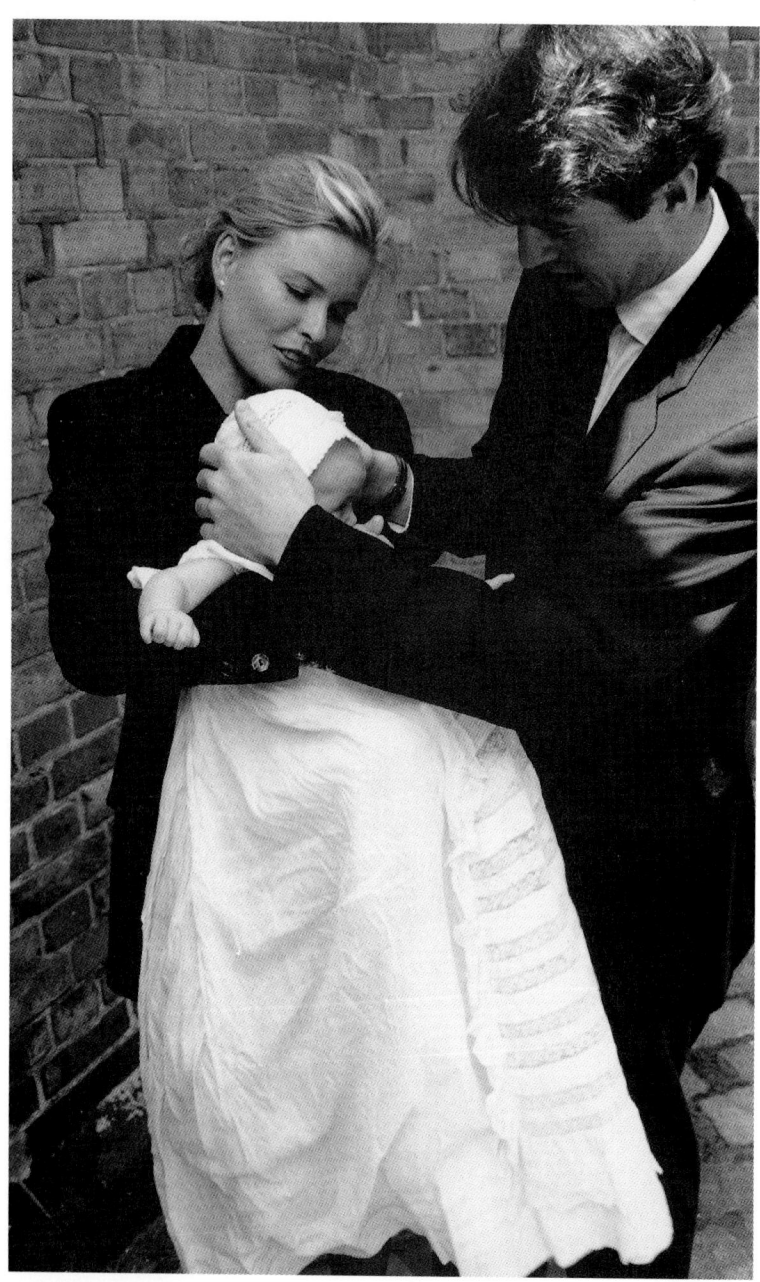

Since becoming parents, my husband and I have developed an even deeper bond than before. But there are certainly tough moments, too!

At other times you'll feel as if you're winging it. You'll be exhausted and anxious, and you'll wonder how you're ever going to pull this off. While it's true I never loved my husband as much as I did after we had our first baby, Julia, sometimes I would look at him lying there fast asleep at 3:00 in the morning, while I got up for the fifth feeding of the night, and think, "Who are you?!" And although I was proud of my body, which had proved itself capable of carrying and sustaining life, sometimes I felt terrible about the way I looked—especially when I would catch a glimpse of my still-ballooning belly in the mirror.

When I gave birth to Julia, who is now three, I realized how unprepared I was for what lay ahead. I was stunned to realize that no one had really ever shared their true stories about how painful it was to give birth, let alone how hard it is to be a new mother. Even my own mother seems to have forgotten that it was anything but easy to have me and raise me, and she raised me by herself.

I started modeling when I was eighteen, and I traveled throughout Europe by myself when I was still a teenager. When I was twenty I moved to the States where I worked for Elizabeth Arden and Revlon, modeled for *Sports Illustrated*, and became a United Nations Children's Fund (UNICEF) spokesperson, so it's not like I'm not used to working long hours, getting by on very little sleep, and feeling overwhelmed (trust me—modeling is glamorous only when the job is done). And I had always had to stay in really good shape, especially when I was posing in next to nothing for *Sports Illustrated* swimsuit issues. You know those models who say they pig out on potato chips and chocolate and don't exercise and still look fantastic? Well, I'm certainly not one of them!

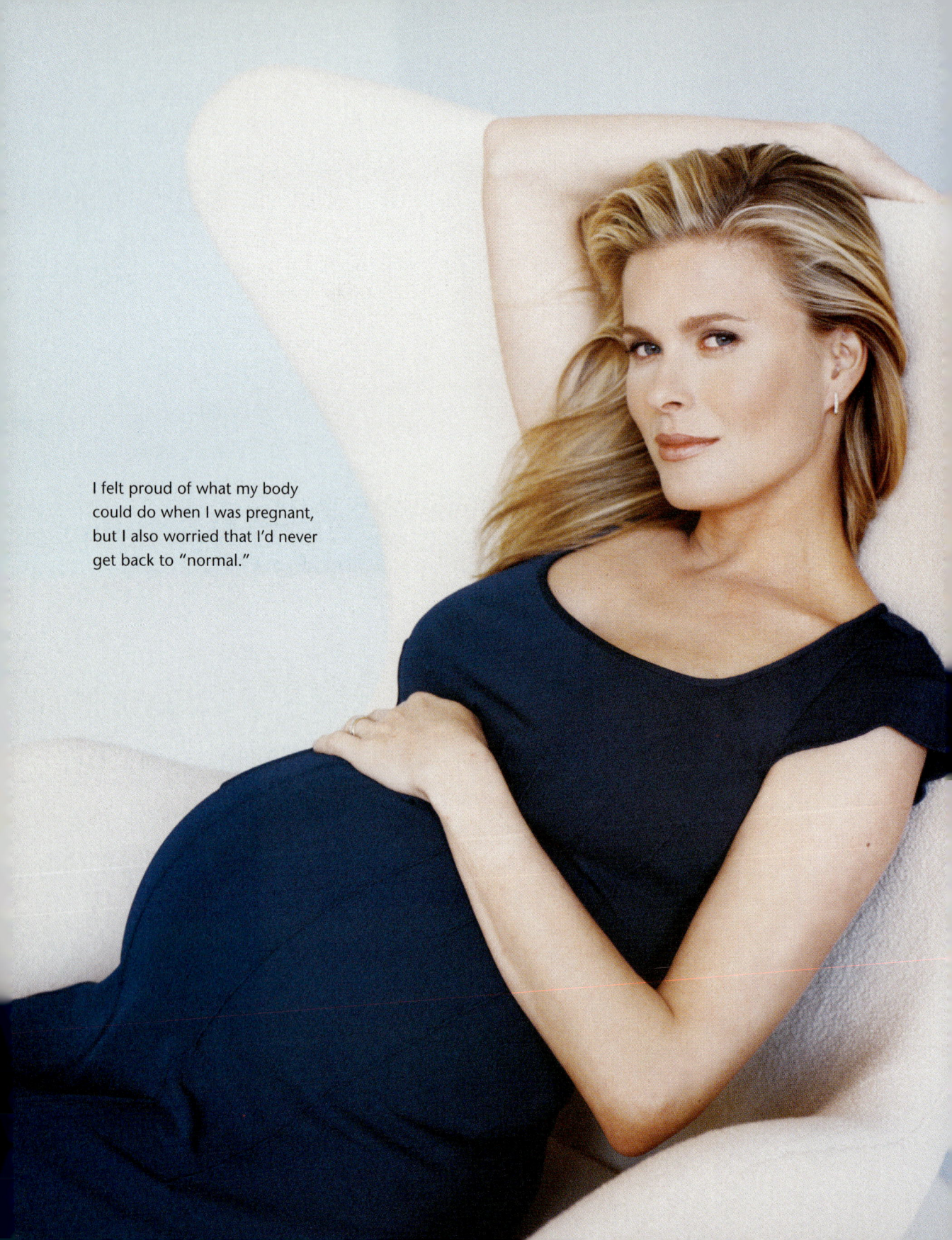

I felt proud of what my body could do when I was pregnant, but I also worried that I'd never get back to "normal."

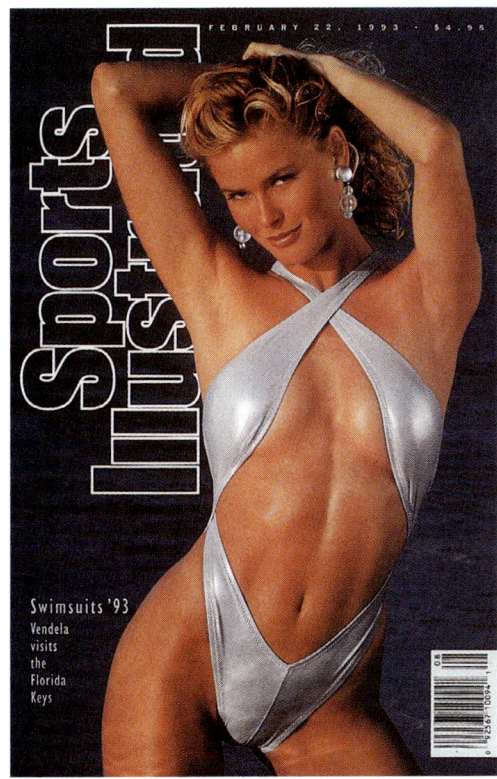

My *Sports Illustrated* cover. I definitely had to work to get into shape for that! (Curto Paolo/*Sports Illustrated*)

But as hard as I had worked over the years and as much as I had had to sweat to get in shape, nothing prepared me for the work and sweat of caring for an infant, my husband, and myself.

Even though I look back on having my first child and realize I had it relatively easy since she slept a lot—until she started getting teeth, when the hell started—I was still constantly late to appointments and feeling like I couldn't get my act together. The first appointment I had scheduled was when she was ten days old, and I was stunned—especially as a formerly punctual person—that I was an hour and a half late, and I still hadn't showered. (It's gotten better since.)

Introduction

The biggest surprise, though, was my discovery that while my close girlfriends were eager to share the high points of their mothering days and would sometimes admit to being sleep-deprived, they would seldom talk openly about those times when they felt like they had no idea what they were doing. If we're not eager to confess to feeling bad about ourselves on good days, we sure don't want to talk about our lives when we have applesauce caked in our hair and bags under our eyes.

I remember walking down the street with my first baby, looking at other mothers and thinking, "What do they know that I don't? Why do they look like they have it so together?" Mothers don't walk up to each other and say, "Well, it took me two hours to get out the door this morning, and even then I was wearing two different socks. How about you?" Instead, we just smile and pass each other by, imagining that other women are somehow gifted in ways we never will be.

We're brought up on beautiful images of mothers looking like the Madonna, all serene and peaceful, and sometimes you're sure to feel that way. But other times I feel as if I'm the only mother in the world who's having a hard time—even if it's doing something as simple as getting my babies dressed to go outside (how do babies know to spit up at the precise second you finish putting them in their clothes?). It's hard to get used to the idea that you're not the earth mother you had fantasized about being when you were pregnant—at least not when your breasts are leaking milk or your baby is screaming in the middle of the restaurant and everyone is giving you dirty looks.

I remember getting ready to leave the hospital after giving birth the first time, and when the nurse handed me Julia, I

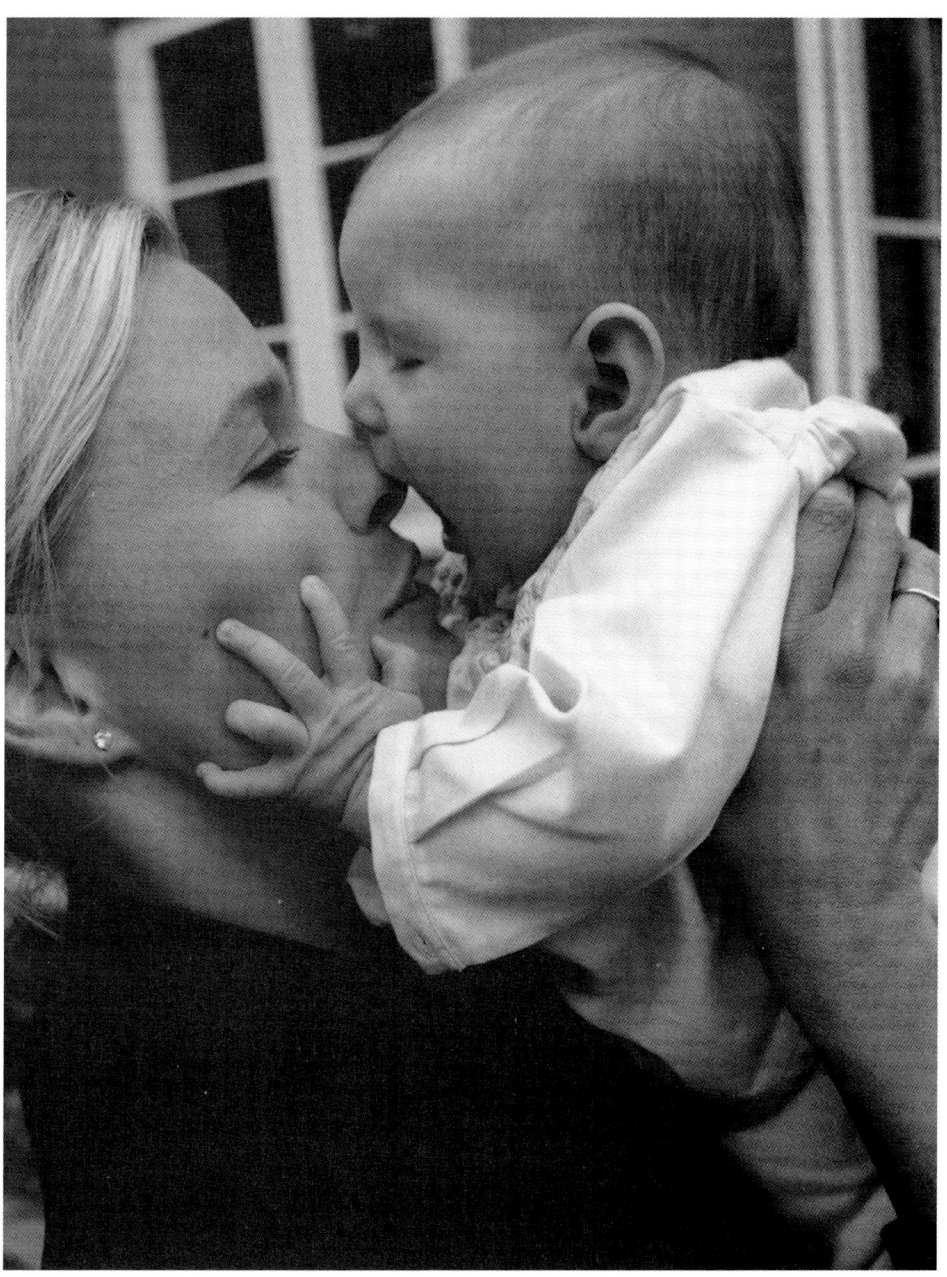

Although I loved being a mother right away, I had no idea how to take care of a baby *and* myself.

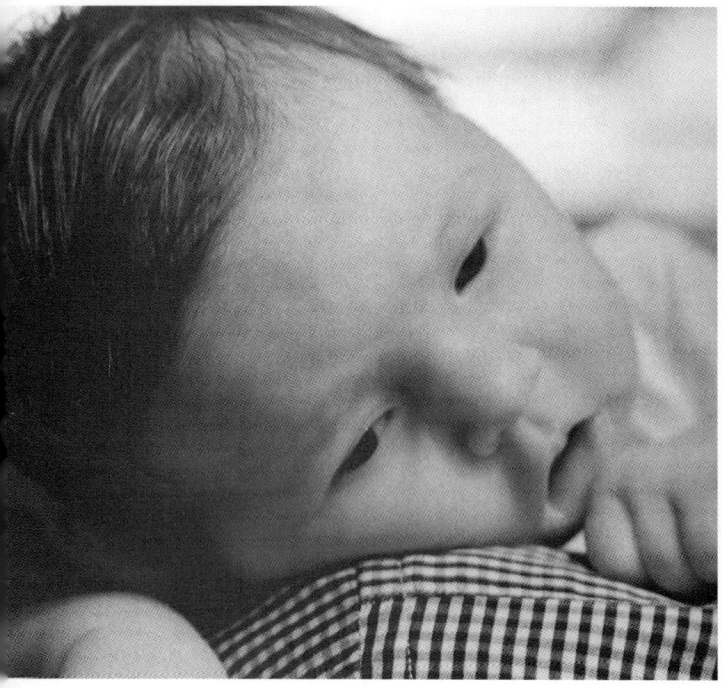

Sometimes it's scary to realize that you are responsible for this new little person.

thought, "Wait! There's been a terrible mistake! I have no idea what I'm doing!" It was even weirder to find myself frightened because I had bonded so fast with her; I hadn't expected a minute of anything but bliss.

Well, if it was a mistake, it was the best one that's ever happened to me, but I wasn't wrong about the second part—I *didn't* have any idea what I was doing. I remember standing at the crib looking down at her sleeping. I felt so lonely and scared, and I thought, "What are we supposed to do now?" At the hospital, there was this warm environment and people to ask for everything, but now suddenly I was on my own.

There I was, responsible for this new life, and I wasn't even sure how I was supposed to live *my* life, never mind know how to breast-feed or read the mind of an infant (I still haven't figured out that last part).

I was very lucky in that I had experts to give me help: Because of my work as a UNICEF spokesperson, I was educated about breast-feeding. And in Sweden, there's a very big

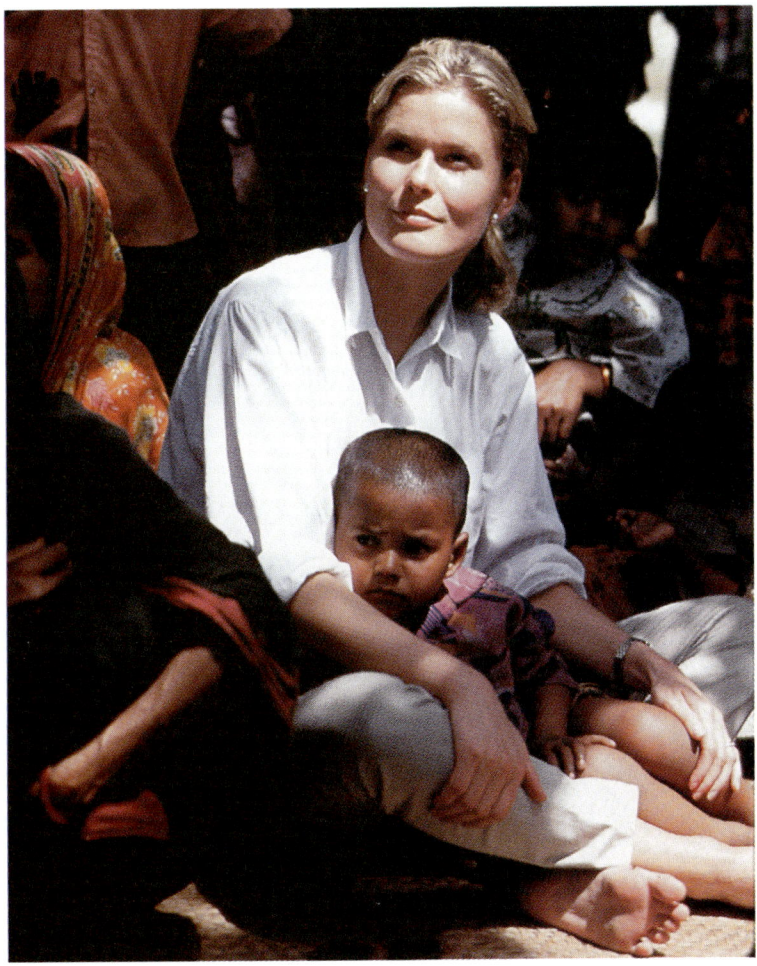

As a spokesperson for UNICEF, I was able to express my love for children even before I had my own.

focus on breast-feeding; it's not only accepted, it's almost forced on you. (I remember feeling like a loser one night when I went into the pharmacy asking for formula and the woman behind the counter said, "Don't you know it's better to breast-feed?" I was going away for work and didn't feel like sitting there and pumping for days, but the woman was so aggressive and angry I ended up not buying the formula!)

In terms of my body, because I had had to get into tip-top shape in the past, I already had an amazing personal trainer, Sean Kelleher. I promise I will pass along all of his best tips!

Needless to say, between my sage advisers and plain old experience, I was a bit better prepared for the arrival of my second child, Hannah. Not that it was easy—after all, having one child doesn't make you an expert at having children, it simply makes you an expert at having *that* child. But this time around, I knew what it would take to get myself back on track. I had figured out how to get all the balls in the air and only drop them occasionally. Most important, I knew exactly what I had to do to make my return to life as a new mom as easy as possible.

I accepted that, while many things seemed beyond my control, there were things I could do for myself that would make me feel more in control, more powerful, and—most vital—like a better mom. While the reality of being a new mom is that your life will never be the same, it can be better than you ever imagined.

Shortly after I first gave birth I was depressed about having gained so much weight, and I thought I would never be able to lose it again. That was really scary, especially since my job is dependent on looking a certain way. But by learning to exercise correctly and eat right, I'm happy with my body

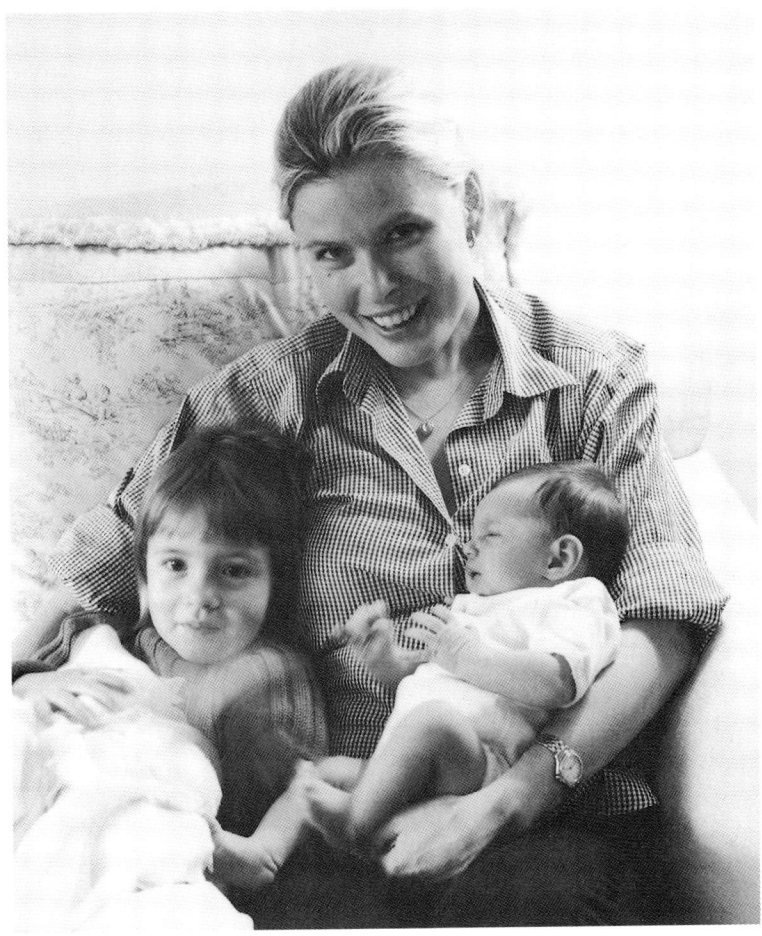

When my second daughter, Hannah, arrived, the adjustment was easier because I knew what to expect—from myself if not from her!

again. In fact, I'm even happier, because I'm so proud that it was able to produce two lives! (I'm not sure my agency feels the same way, but more on that later.)

I was also nervous that my relationship with my husband would never recover from the sudden lack of private time together. In addition, I wasn't sure my husband could learn to

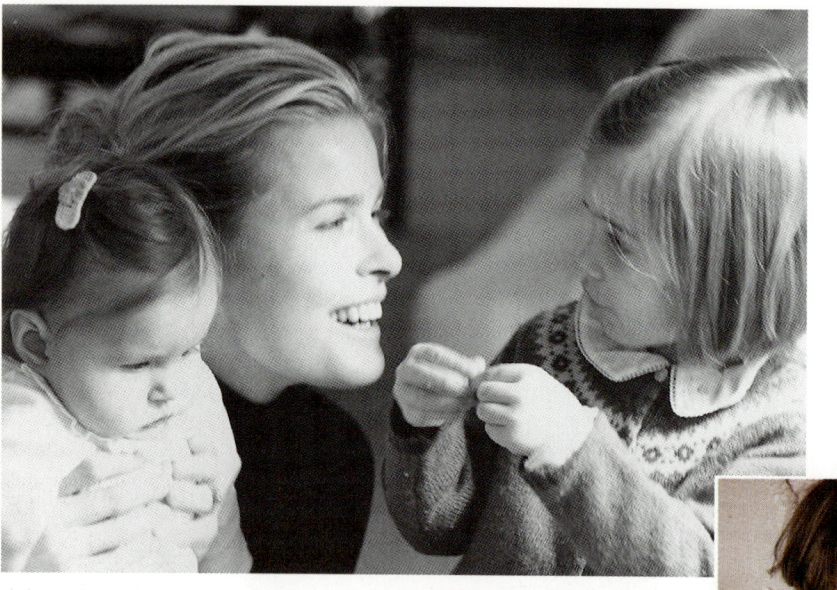
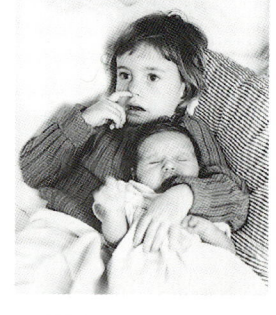
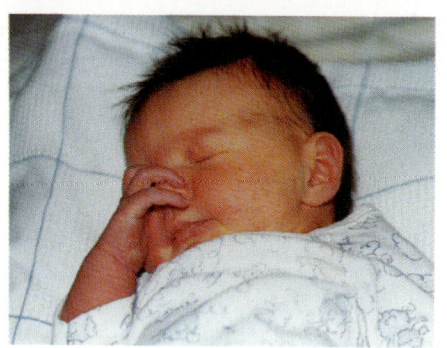
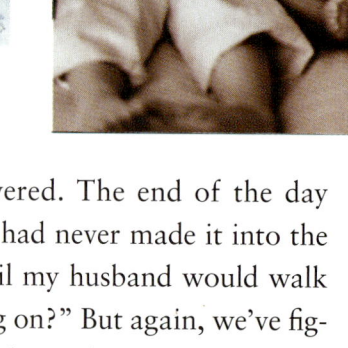

My personal photo album, from the girls' earliest days.

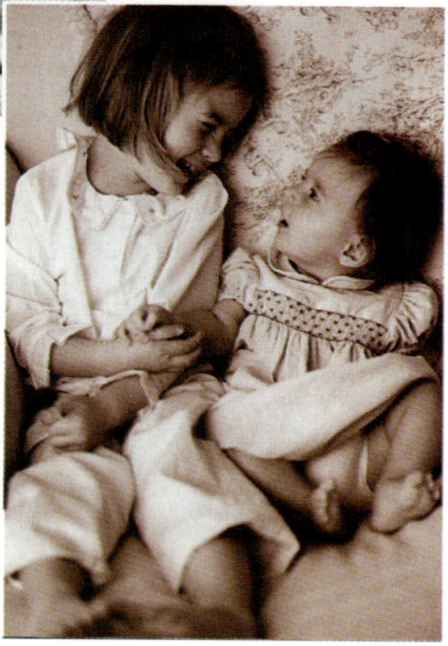

live with a wife who never showered. The end of the day would come and I would realize I had never made it into the bath. I wouldn't even know it until my husband would walk in the door and say, "What is going on?" But again, we've figured out some tricks to make our relationship even stronger—tricks I'll pass on to you so you don't have to learn them the hard way, as I did.

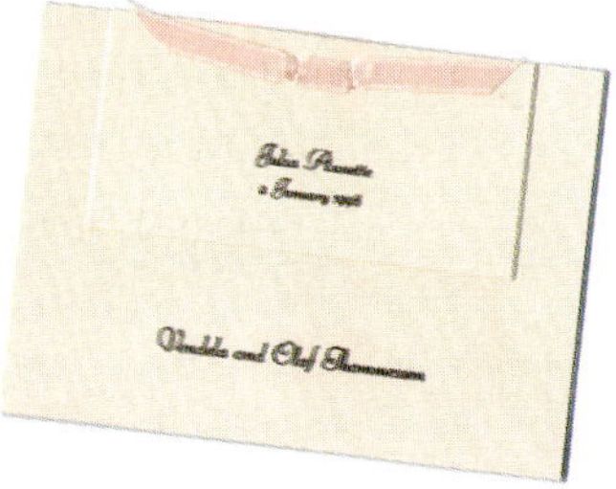

This book will serve as an honest guide to living your first few months as a mom. It will

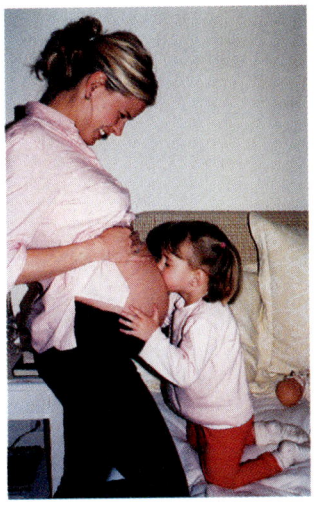 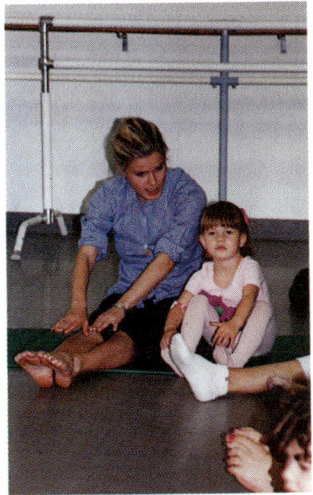 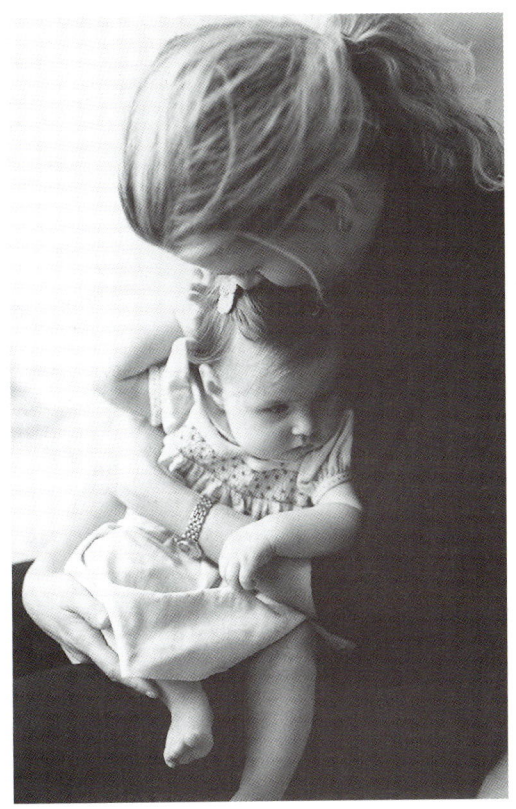

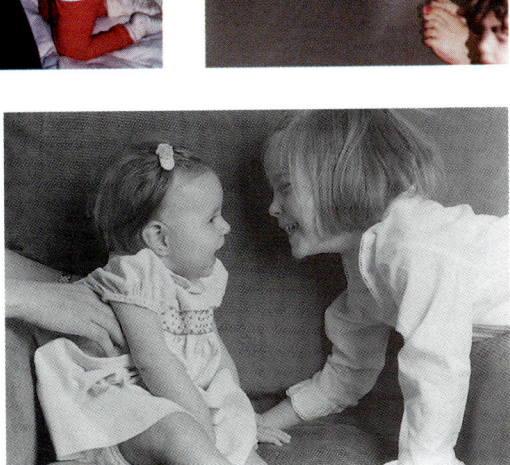

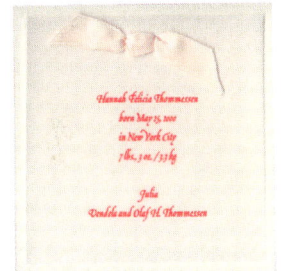

remind you that any experience you're having, believe me, you're not the first one living through it!

When I had my children, I sometimes felt so isolated, especially when I couldn't comfort my crying baby, or I'd be convinced I'd never get rest again or be able to wear anything but maternity clothes for the rest of my life. This book will assure you that every mother has dark days of thinking these things, that there are ways to help you through those times, and that—here's the key—those dark days end!

Introduction

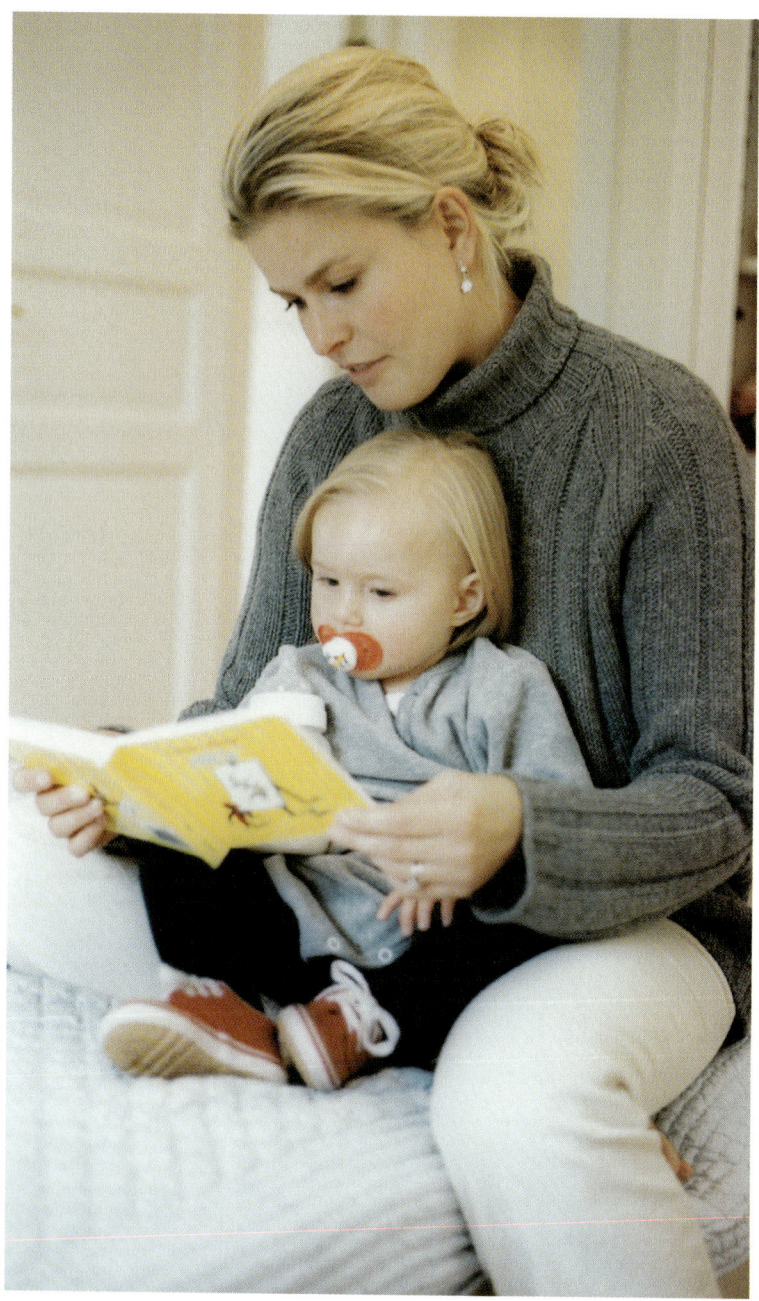

Realize that you are stronger and more beautiful than ever now that you are a mother.

As a new mother, you have enough to worry about, but there are some things you shouldn't have any anxiety about: in as little as three to six months, you *can* get back into shape. You will feel proud of yourself. You will feel confident and in control and beautiful—even when spit-up has become your newest accessory. And you will thrive as a mother and a wife.

This is your chance to realize that you're stronger than you've ever known, more beautiful than you've ever hoped, and a better mother than you ever thought possible. Sound impossible? Actually, it's not hard at all. And you can accomplish all of these things with applesauce in your hair, dressed in mismatched socks, and functioning on no sleep. Trust me—if I've done it twice, it can't be that hard!

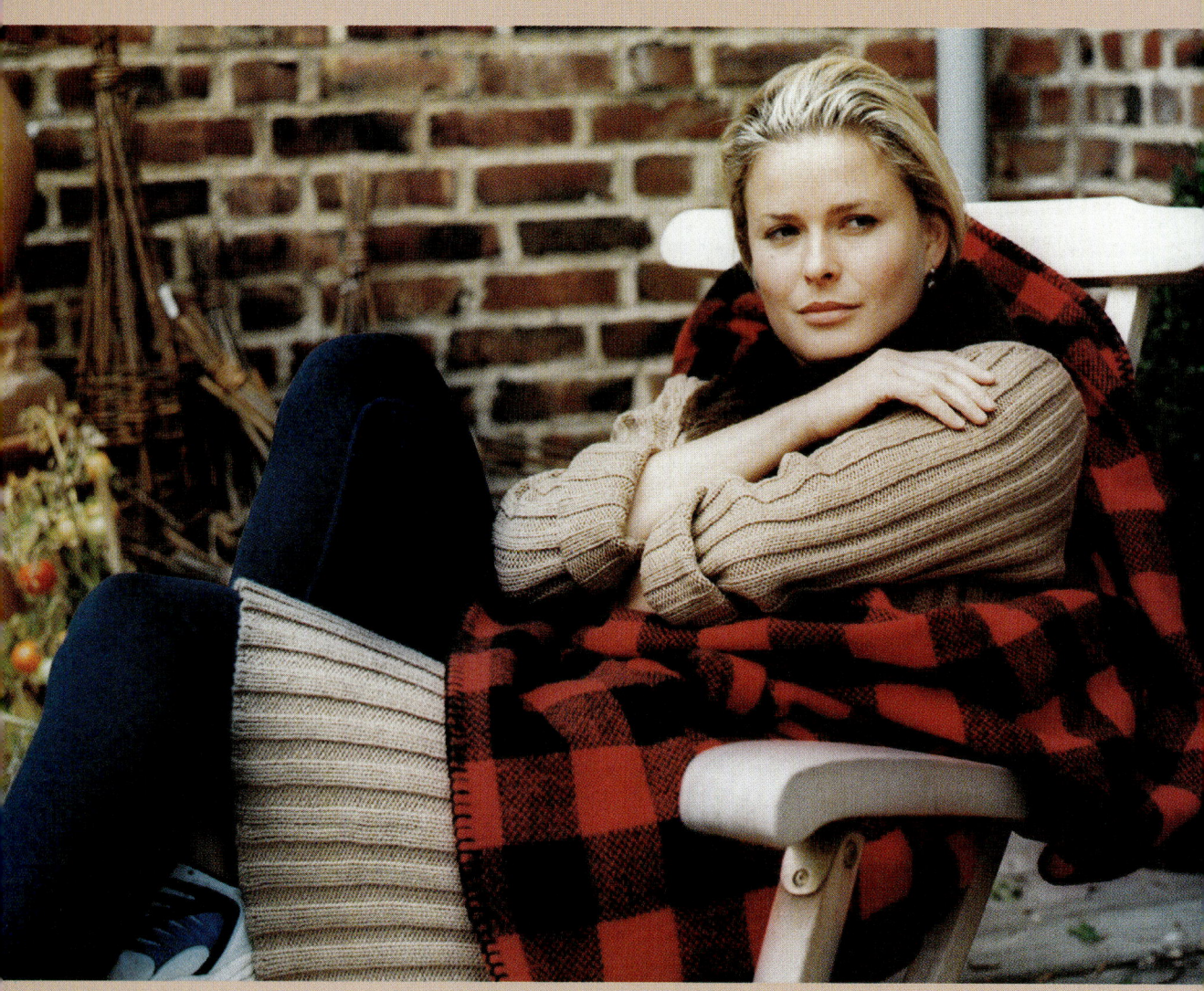

PART ONE

Emotional Rescue

What to expect and how to deal with your new life and an avalanche of new feelings

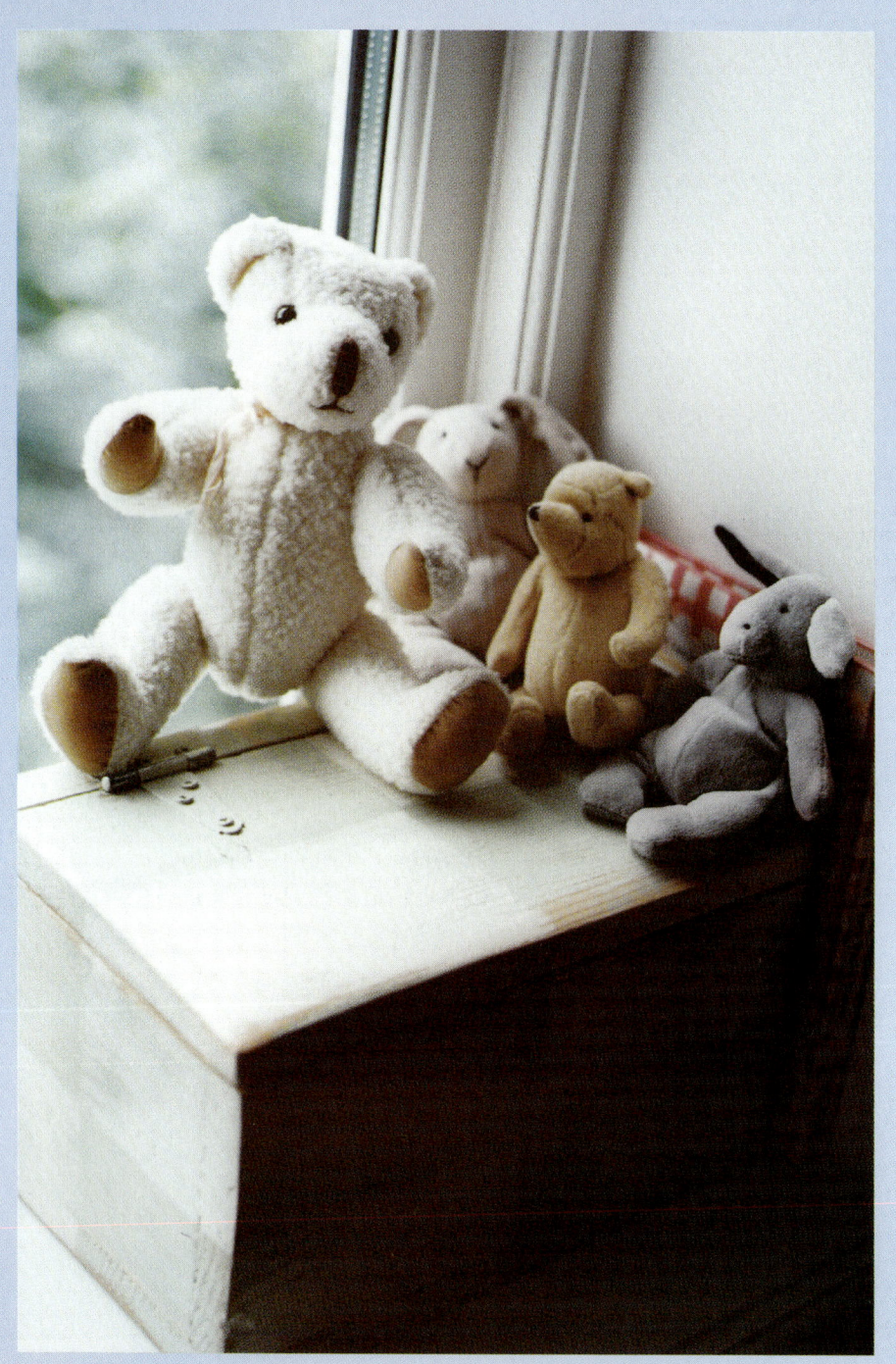

1

Hello Hormones, Good-Bye Serenity!

I always knew that I wanted to have children, and after my husband and I had been married about a year, we decided it was time to start trying. At the time, I was busy modeling and pursuing an acting career. I had some reservations about how I could be a mom and still be able to hold down a frantic work schedule, but I figured we'd be trying for at least a year, and that would give me plenty of time to figure out how, exactly, I was going to continue to work and be a mother and a wife. You can imagine how surprised we were when I got pregnant right away.

I had a feeling I had to make changes in my life if I wanted children, so I made some tough decisions. I put my acting career on hold. Because my husband's business involves a lot of traveling throughout Europe, I left L.A. to live with him in New York. The move would have been an emotional time no matter what, but it certainly didn't help that through it all I was having incredible mood swings because of my pregnancy. It was a pretty tough time of making adjustments.

Although I had made these decisions I don't think I really knew ahead of time how much of my old life I was going to give up to become a mother. That knowledge comes gradually. Plus, it's so much easier not to feel like you're making sacrifices when you have your beautiful baby in front of you.

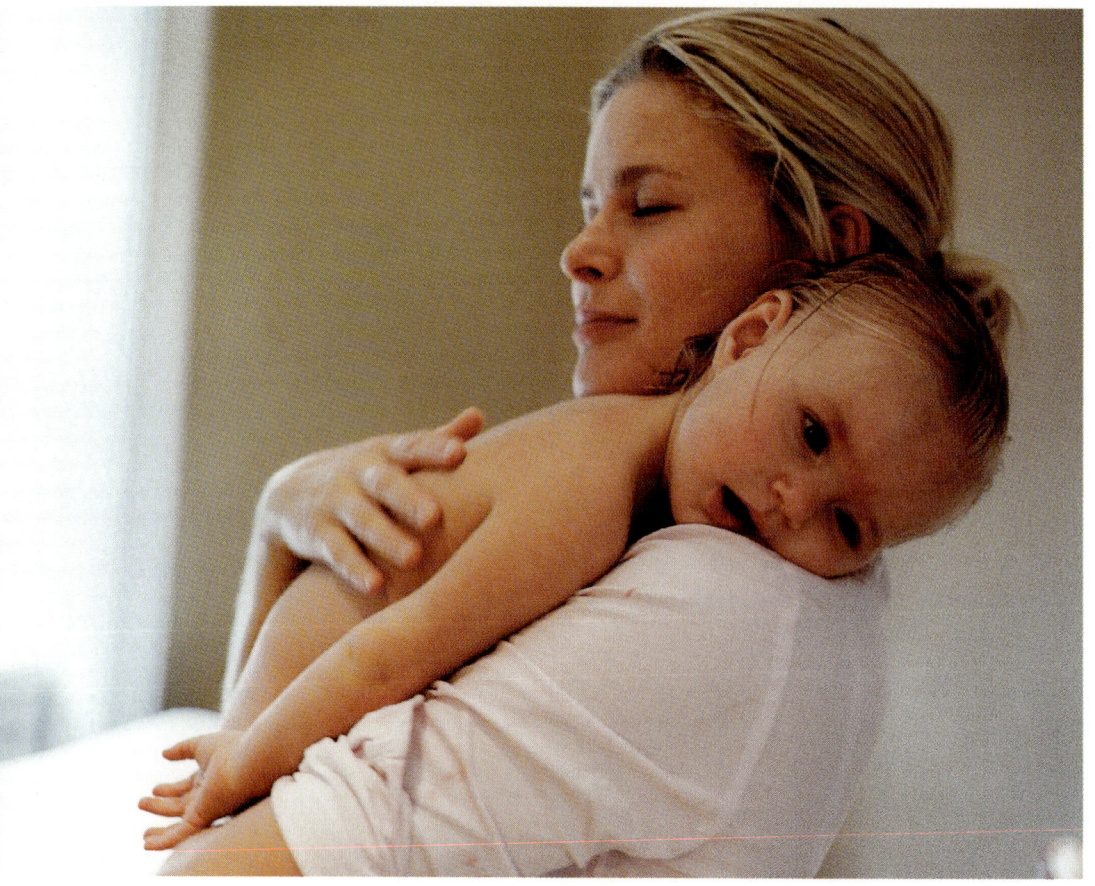

I fell in love with my baby even before she was born, but I still had hormonal swings after her birth.

Well, it's a *little* easier, anyway. I was very, very lucky in that I, like many other women, fell in love with my baby before she even came out into the world. And the second I gave birth and the nurse put Julia in my arms, I felt like I was a part of a miracle. But I have to admit that I still had enormous hormonal swings for the first few months after I'd given birth.

The emotional roller coaster can be scary. Most of the time you're happier than you've ever been, but then suddenly your brain is skipping all over the place. And no one is honest about it. Women don't sit around having coffee saying, "Sometimes, for the first time in my life, I think I'm losing my mind."

Since I knew that it was the hormones making me feel like a crazy person when I gave birth to Hannah, my second child, I was OK. But the first time, with Julia, there were times when I was really frightened. Julia would start screaming, and I would start sweating and saying, "What am I doing wrong?" I'd get all worked up about it, and she'd keep crying, and pretty soon I'd be crying too.

Looking back I can see that my anxiety was ridiculous because of course all the crying (on my baby's part, anyway) was because Julia was hungry or tired. Now I know that, and when Hannah cried, I would try feeding her or putting her to sleep, and it almost always worked. (Obviously, when your child is sick, this all goes out the window; you're both back to getting no sleep and feeling crazy.)

It didn't help that I was feeling like my career was over. I felt lonely and left out. I felt like I was misunderstood and that even my husband didn't know me. I also felt like all the sacrificing that was being done was being done on my part, some-

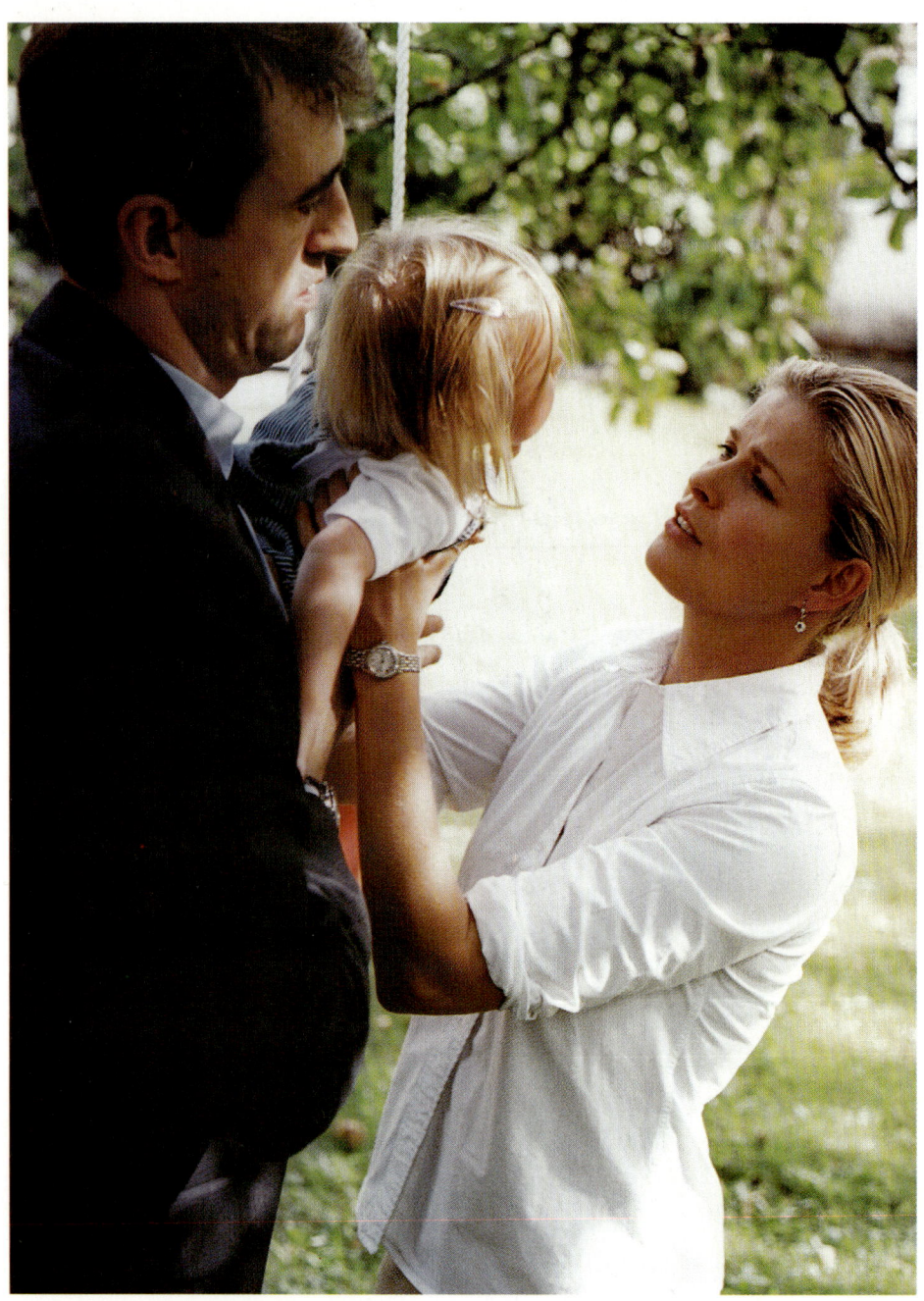

Even the best fathers sometimes need reminding of all that you are going through.

thing that is true for most women. The reality is it's impossible to be parents unless one of you is there most of the time, making the children your first priority. Most of the time, that's fine, but sometimes it can feel totally unfair.

Still, in retrospect, I do see that it was impossible for Olaf to understand what I was going through, since even I didn't fully understand it. Sometimes, I wish that husbands could go through a similar experience at the same time.

When I would have a hard afternoon with Julia, the last thing I wanted to do was bother my husband at work. I thought, "He's going to think he's married to a crazy woman." I didn't want him to worry that I couldn't take care of our child. In fact, talking to him turned out to be the best thing I could have done. He would remind me that I was a wonderful mother and that while I might have felt nuts for a moment, I wasn't suddenly becoming a raving lunatic. Simply hearing the words come out of my mouth also made me feel less nuts. Things sound so much less scary when they're said out loud.

Once I was done reminding my husband that my hormones were out of control, I'd remind myself. Maybe you'll be really lucky and never have any doubts or panics or hard times. But if you do, just remind yourself that it's going to pass, and that part of the reason you're feeling out of control emotionally is that your body is zinging with hormones.

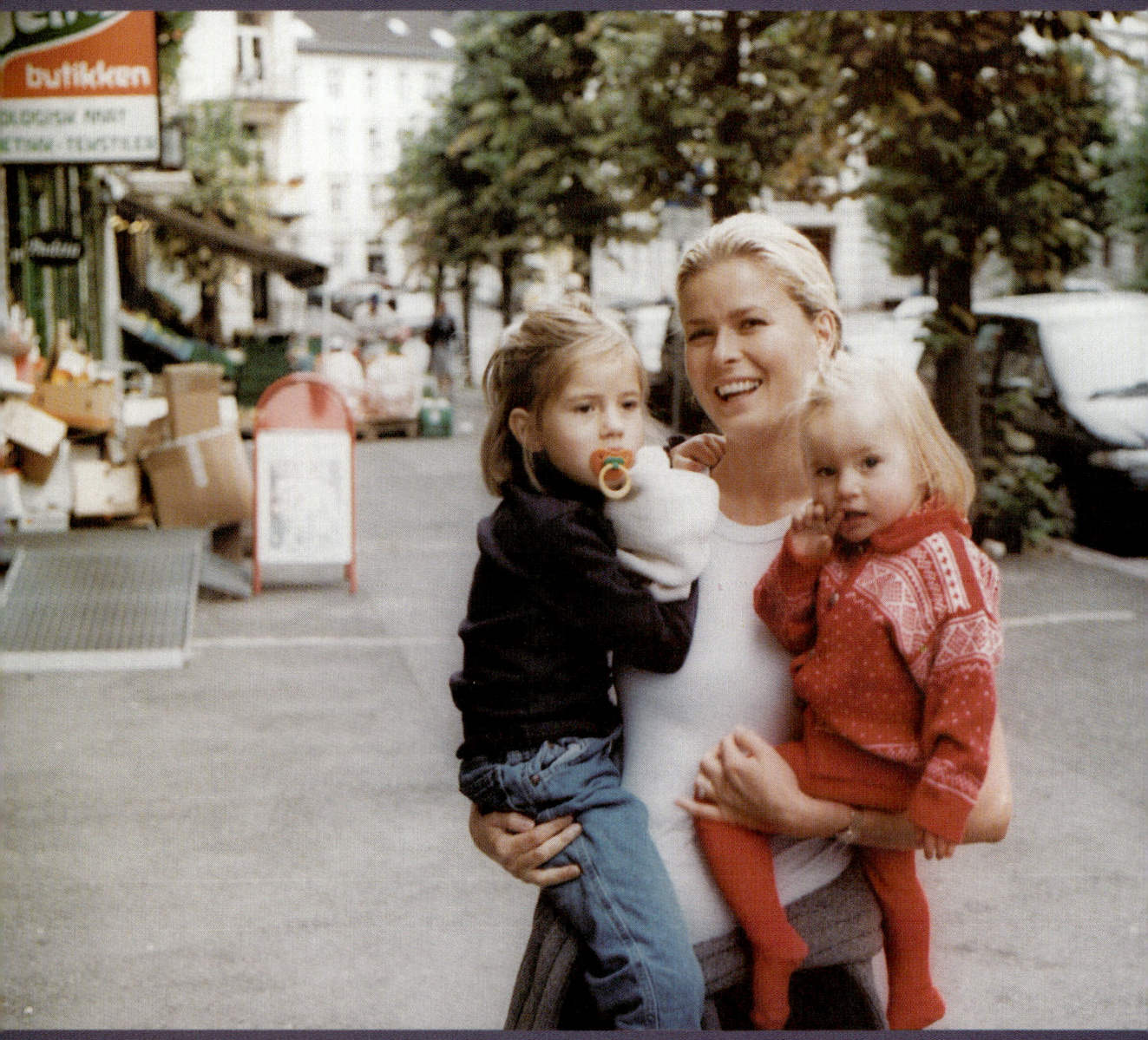

2

The Hardest Job You'll Ever Love

I'm convinced that women forget what it's like to have infants. Or they remember just the wonderful parts, of which there are many.

When I had just had my babies, I would call my mother to tell her that I was up all night with one of my children, or that I had had a hard day, and she would say, "Every day with you was a joy. You were so easy." And I'd think, "Why am I different? Why did I get children who aren't so easy?" You can feel guilty that somehow you're not pulling off this thing called motherhood that every woman is supposed to innately know how to do.

Some days when I'm walking down the street with my daughters, someone will stop me and ask, "How are you?" and I'll say, "I'm great," but inside I'm thinking, "Yeah, right, I'm great." Recently, I had to go to a christening, so my daughters and I had to be dressed up. My husband was away on business, and I was trying to get all three of us dressed and out the door. The little one was dressed but started screaming, and then Julia wanted to take her tights off and wear the wrong shoes, and here I was in a pair of panty hose with a run in them and I didn't have another pair. . . . I just had to go into the hallway and scream for a minute. It was one of those moments when I forgot that most days are great, and I was thinking, "I want to cry and I can't even do that!"

Sometimes when you're tired, it can all seem like too much, which is why *you have to learn to cut yourself some slack*. Whatever it is you need to do to blow off some energy without affecting your children, do it! For me, when things really get crazy, the last resort is to step out for a second and have a quick scream in the hallway. (I can only imagine what the neighbors think, but at that point, they are the least of my concerns!)

Happily, most of the time simply taking a deep breath can do the trick. There were some nights when no amount of breast-feeding or rocking could comfort Hannah or Julia, and they would just be so, so sad and frustrated and screaming their heads off. I used to feel like a terrible mom, like I should be able to read their minds at all times, but now I know that there are times when a baby just needs to cry. And there are times when I need to step outside the bedroom door and take a deep breath. (Of course I always make sure the child is in a safe place, like her crib, and I'm only gone for thirty seconds.)

At first I felt like a terrible mother for having to step out of the room, but I realized that my anxiety was only compounding my children's anxiety. (On the other hand, I feel like a terrible mother no matter what I do, sometimes. That guilt thing is awful and powerful.) But no child is going to die if you go out of the room for a few minutes and take some time for yourself. In fact, by taking a two-second time-out for

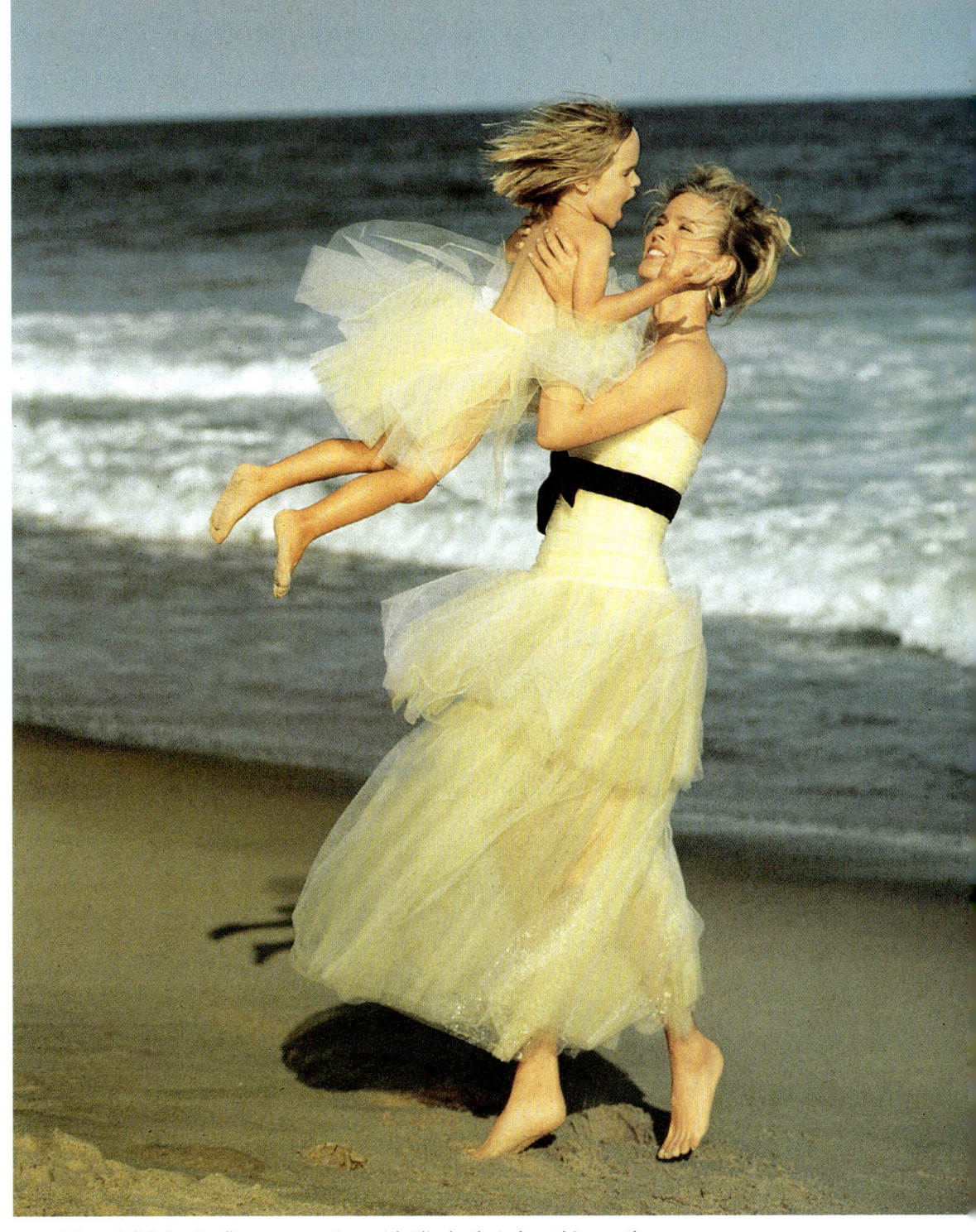

When I did the Sunflower campaign with Elizabeth Arden, this was the closest I came to knowing what it was like to have a child. The reality is decidedly less glamorous! (Copyright © Patrick Demarchelier, Inc.)

The Hardest Job You'll Ever Love

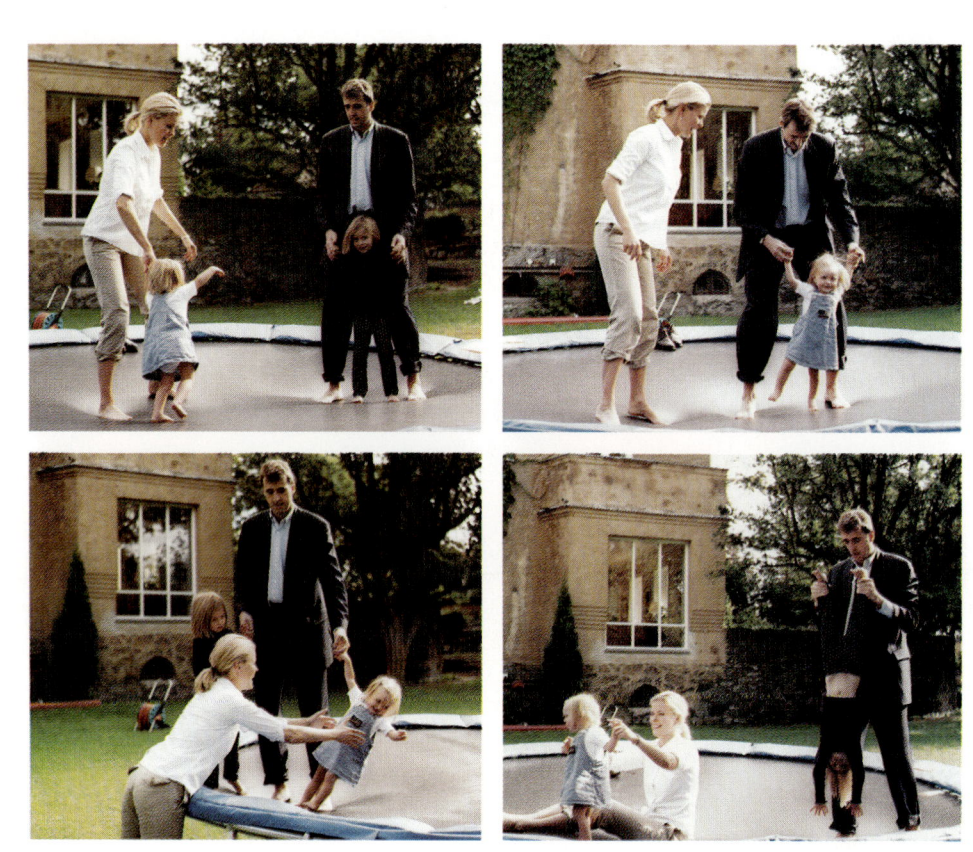

Sometimes the whole family can blow off steam together with some physical activity. It really helps!

myself, I was able to calm down and recenter myself so that when I went back into the room there was only one upset person in there instead of two.

Another trick that I'm terrible at but I hope you can be better with is asking for help. When I was living in New York and my husband was traveling I would be up all night with the kids, and I would find myself finally getting all the kids into one bed, with myself wrapped around their feet like a dog.

That's when you really need to ask a friend to spend the night or take one of the kids for a while. For my part, I think it was hard for me to feel like I was falling apart, and I didn't want to admit it to anyone. I also wanted to be there for both of my children 100 percent, and I felt that, somehow, if I had had some help I'd be short-changing them. Now I realize they would have benefited from getting some attention from someone who had had two hours of sleep rather than none. I had to learn to accept my limitations, to grab sleep whenever I could, and most important to *plan on not planning*.

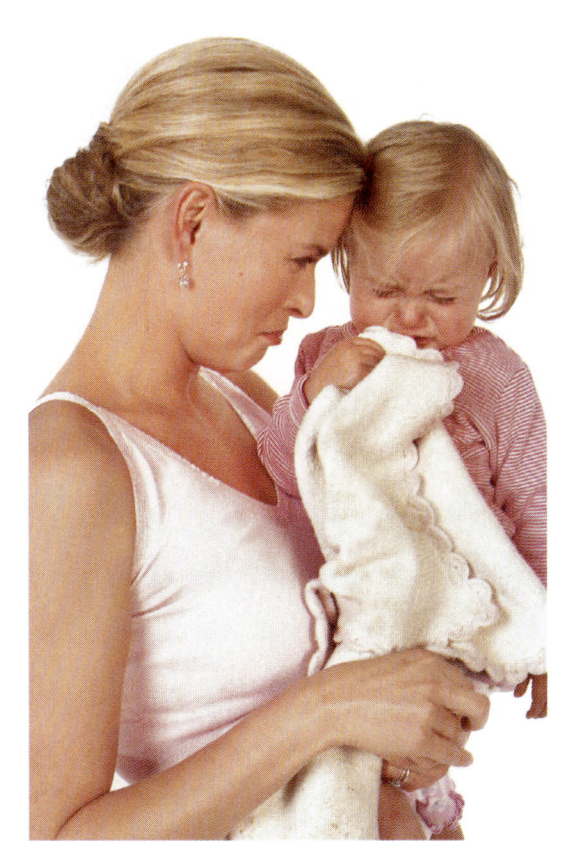

It's important to remember that all babies cry sometimes. Just take a deep breath, go outside, and scream—whatever helps.

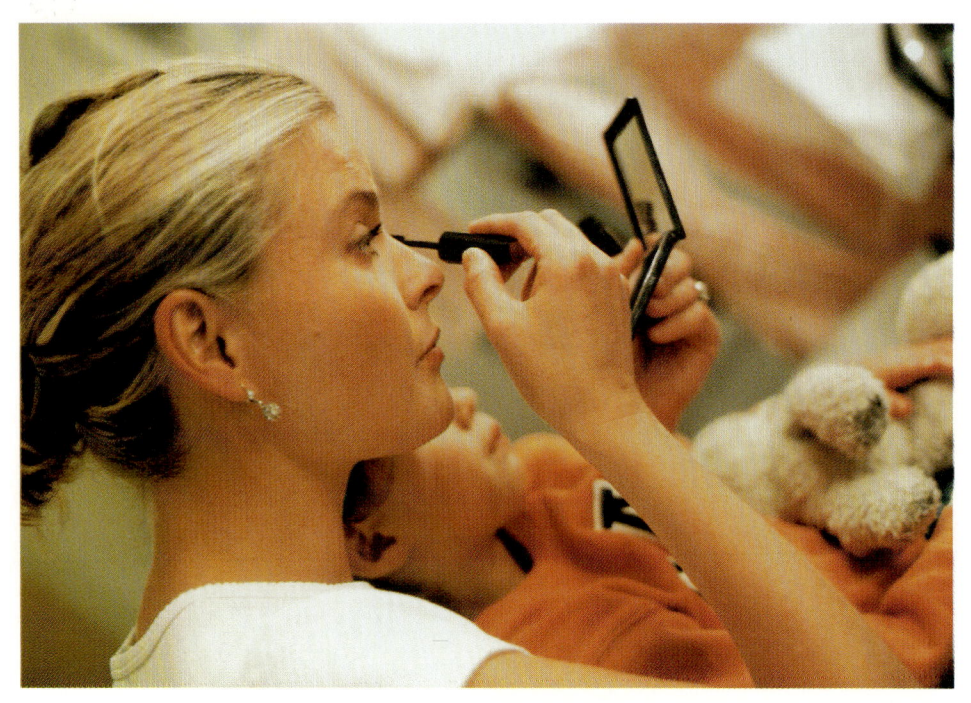

I've learned to accept that being a good mom can mean compromising in other areas. I've even had to bring my daughters along on a shoot. Here Julia cuddled on my lap while I put the final touches on my makeup.

There will be many times when you won't have the ability to put yourself first—even for a minute. Before I became a mom, I was a fanatical list keeper. I felt that if I didn't accomplish everything on that day's list, I had somehow failed.

Well, let me tell you—throw out those lists and you'll spare yourself many a moment of frustration! (However, the compulsive part of me wants to add that I still make lists in my head in order to stay on a strict routine, which helps my anal side keep it together—especially with two kids.)

I think it's really important to give yourself ways to feel like you've accomplished things, but remember—an infant doesn't understand your need to stick to an agenda. Recently I was on my way to a job when I got a call that Julia was sick, so I called work and said, "I can't come. I have to go home." I was really lucky that that was an option, but the moral is there's no point in making a schedule for yourself that you're going to feel bad about having to cancel—because, inevitably, you will! Just remember that sometimes being a really good mom means falling short in other areas.

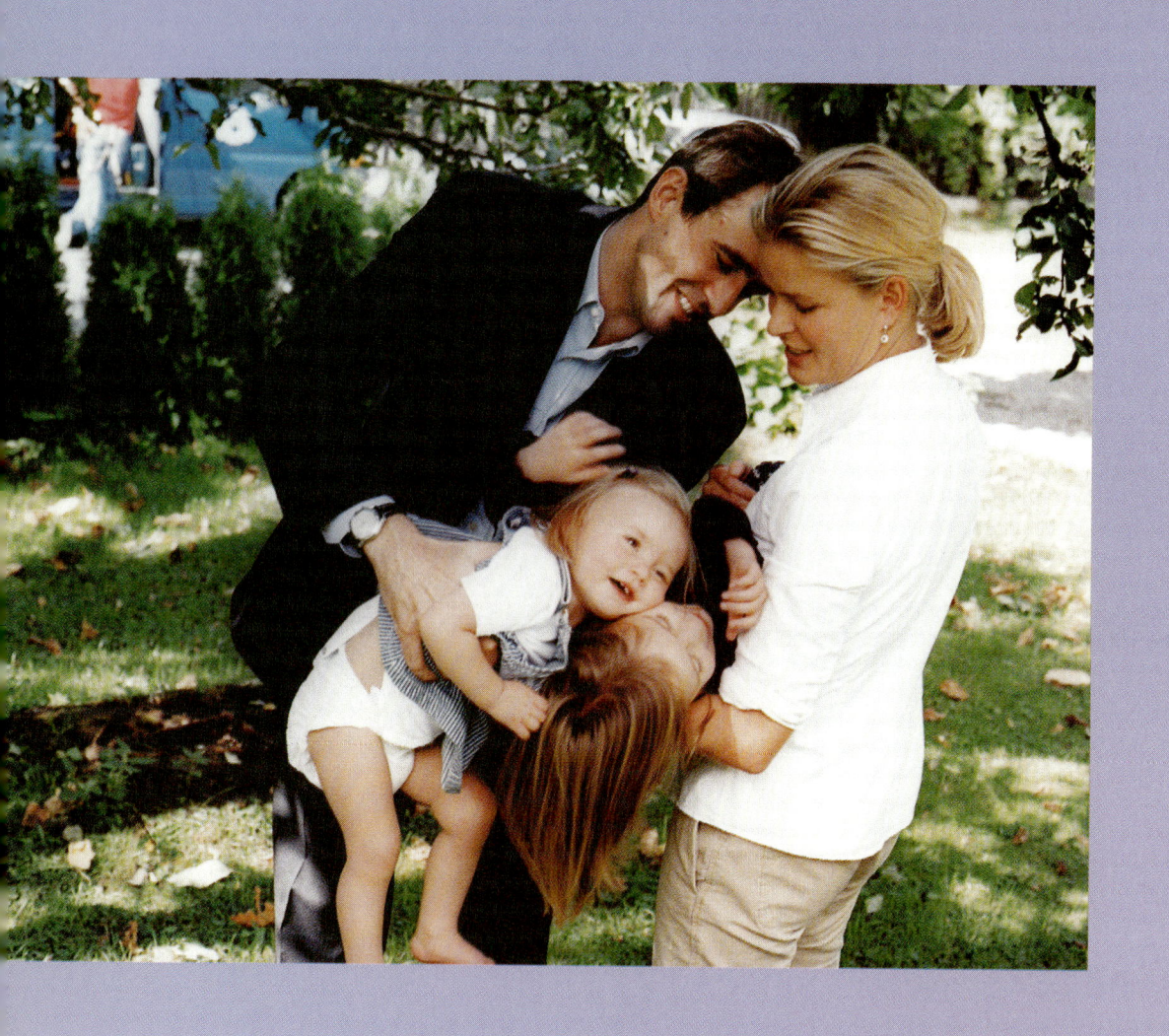

3

A Marriage of Minds

Both people in a couple need to be aware that a new baby brings a lot of life changes, and they should talk about those changes as much as they can.

Right around the time I gave birth to Hannah my husband started a new job that involved even more traveling than he did before. Four months later I realized that we had never really had a chance to talk about what exactly his new job entailed. That night, after we put the kids to bed, we turned off the phone and the television, opened a bottle of wine, and sat down on the couch to talk. It was the first time since I had had Hannah that we both remembered that the two of us had a relationship that needed to be maintained, too, and I vowed to make some changes. (Again, I emphasize that I was the one making the changes. I think that, unfortunately, it's often up to the woman to recognize when a situation isn't working, and that means she is often the one to make the appropriate sacrifices to change it.)

Some of the changes we agreed on were incredibly easy to make. I had simply been too tired to think of them, let alone execute them. Let's call them the One Rules.

- Once a week, for one hour, that's your time together. It's lovely if you're able to schedule a night out together, but sometimes that might be aiming too high. That entails hiring a baby-sitter, who might cancel, or one of you might have to work late, and the entire evening is blown.

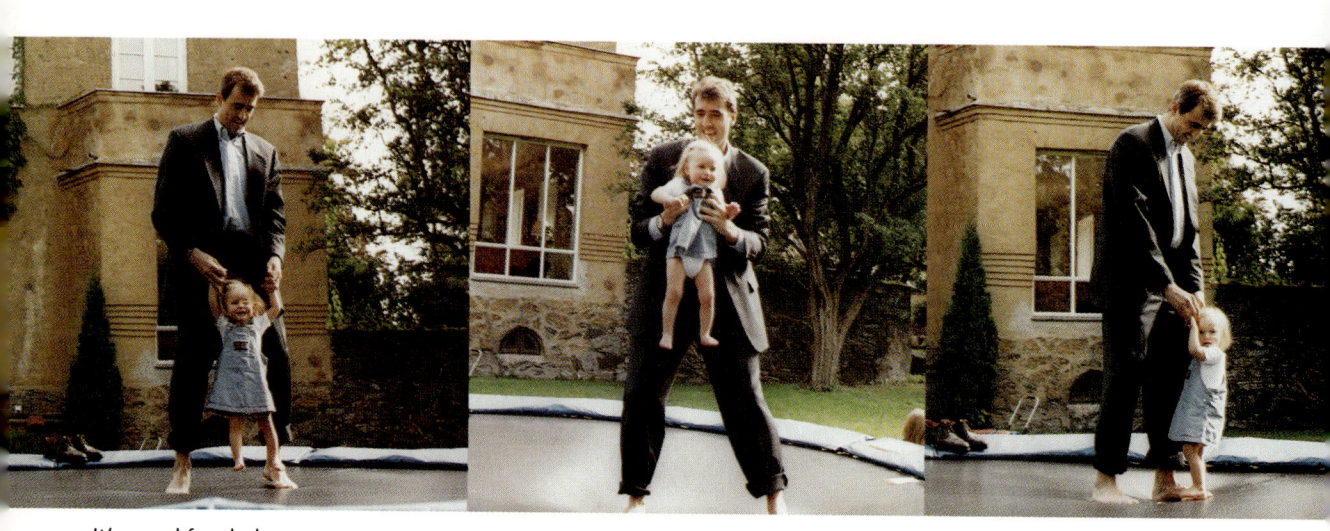

It's good for dads to have some alone time with the kids. (It's good for moms too.)

But if you schedule an hour at home after your children are asleep, your chances of sticking to it are much, much better. And who knows? Maybe that hour can stretch into several. (That said, there will be nights you may not have the energy to talk for longer than an hour—don't beat yourself up about it.)

My husband and I designate one evening a week when we think we'll be done working at a normal time. We make no other plans. We let the answering machine get the calls, and we just hang out. We also try to talk about things other than the children for that allotted period of time.

There's no pressure to get dressed up or be romantic—the focus is just on talking. And the remarkable thing is that without the pressures of having to change clothes or act sensual, those usually end up being the most romantic evenings we have. And should they not turn into a real "date," that's fine— no one's disappointed. We've had an hour to catch up and hold hands.

- Once a week, for one hour, it's *his* turn. Don't wait until you're on the brink of getting angry to ask for alone time, and don't feel like you have to have something really important planned to justify time off by yourself.

What I missed the most with infants was time doing nothing. I missed sitting quietly with a cup of coffee in a cafe, I missed having my nails done, I missed going for a walk without a small child trailing me. Tell your husband that for one hour that suits you both, he's in charge of the baby. It's bonding time for them, and it's regrouping time for you.

If you can, keep the time consistent; otherwise, something will come up that makes it impossible. Recently, I really wanted to go have a manicure and some time to myself, and at the last minute, my husband said to our daughter, "Julia, do you want to go with Mommy?" What was I going to say? Julia and I ended up having a great time, but it wasn't what I had in mind, and frankly, Julia and I have plenty of fun times during the day. What I needed was alone time, something my husband is able to have without even thinking about it, whether it's on his ride to work or during his lunch hour.

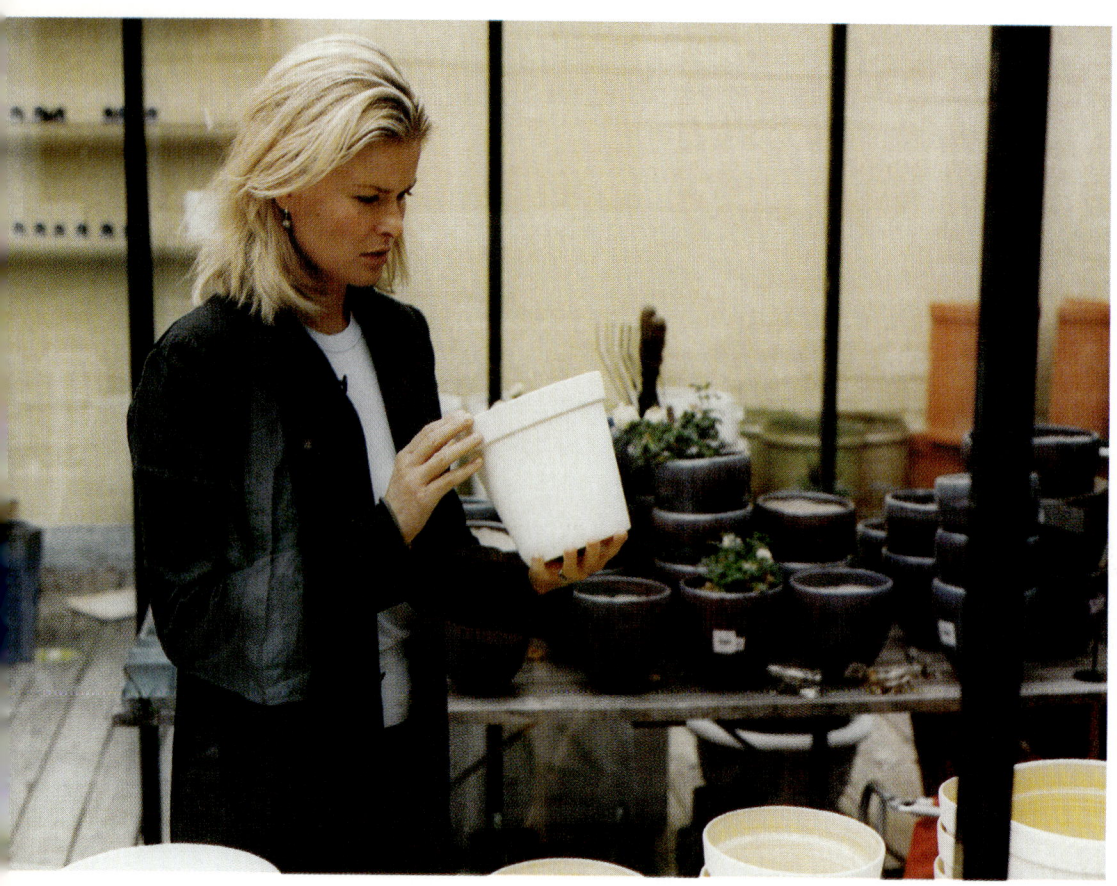

One of my glorious
alone times.

    So mark it on your calendars in indelible ink that from, say, 11 A.M. to 12 P.M. on Saturdays you're disappearing. And then do exactly that. When you come back in the house, you'll no doubt find your husband and child happy in each other's company. Or at least they'll both be thrilled to see you! And you'll be happy to see them, too.

    I learned this lesson the hard way: at one point I became so run down and sick that my doctor threatened to hospitalize me just so I could get some rest; I found it impossible to take to my bed for the day, something my husband would do without thinking twice. I realized that, just as he wouldn't ask my permission to do it, I shouldn't have to either. A mother's job is 24/7, whereas a dad can often feel that he has "put in his time" after a couple of hours.

I think that there's a genetic disposition at work here, as well—men feel comfortable taking, and women feel more comfortable giving. It's difficult to recognize that this can go too far, to the point that the woman is giving more than is healthy. I think it's really important for a couple to try to work together to be a happy family—which involves both of you feeling fulfilled.

- One night a week, he does one feeding. If you have the luxury of not working but your husband is working, it may not make sense for your husband to be sharing nighttime feedings with you. If you're breast-feeding exclusively, as I have with both of my children, it's impossible.

However, it is still possible to share the feeding duties. You and your husband can agree that on Friday or Saturday nights, you'll pump your breast milk (or prepare a bottle of formula), and he'll do the feedings while you sleep in. Not only is this a nice thing for you—that extra few hours of sleep can feel like a miracle!—it's also good for your husband. Often, the father can feel left out when the mom is breast-feeding the baby. This arrangement gives dad and baby an hour of intimate contact usually reserved for mom and baby.

It's ironic that the one thing that made having a baby possible is the one thing you're *really* not likely to feel like doing for a while. Don't panic—I promise your sex drive will come back, but it can be pretty quick to disappear in the first few months.

A Marriage of Minds

After my first child, I really didn't feel like it. You know how you have to wait six weeks after giving birth for the doctor to give you the go-ahead? Well, after Julia, I remember coming home and wondering if I could tell my husband that the doctor had proclaimed I had a rare case of something that would make sex impossible for the immediate future (no such luck!). But when I had Hannah, I was eager for the six weeks to be done. One thing in particular that was weird for me, even though I felt like having sex, was having my husband touch my breasts; I was breast-feeding and I felt as though my breasts weren't sexual anymore. There's just no telling how you're going to feel, so don't beat yourself up for it.

There are some small things you can do to help yourself feel sexy again, even if it's just wearing perfume. After I had Hannah, I guess my body chemistry changed because I suddenly didn't like the way my old perfume smelled on me. So I went out and bought a new one, and when I walked in the door and my husband told me I smelled wonderful, I felt really great. Following my exercise and eating suggestions can also do wonders for your sex drive, since you'll feel good about your body that much faster.

In Sweden people are much more up-front about sexuality and bodies, so it was always talked about—learning to do Keigel exercises, where you squeeze your vaginal muscles as if you're trying to stop peeing midstream, was as appropriate a conversation over a dinner table as what was for dinner. It's really important to do your Keigels; women who do them complain far less often about vaginal stretching and incontinence after giving birth.

The other thing not to underestimate in terms of your sex drive is that you'll not only feel ugly sometimes but also really boring—hardly a turn-on for either of you. My husband never had to give up reading the newspaper in the morning or an interesting novel at night, when I'd be busy trying to feed the children or recovering from the day. It would have been helpful to sit down and talk to him about it—instead of just stewing with rage—and say, "It's Wednesday. It's my day to read the paper, so you give the kids breakfast." It will benefit both of you, believe me.

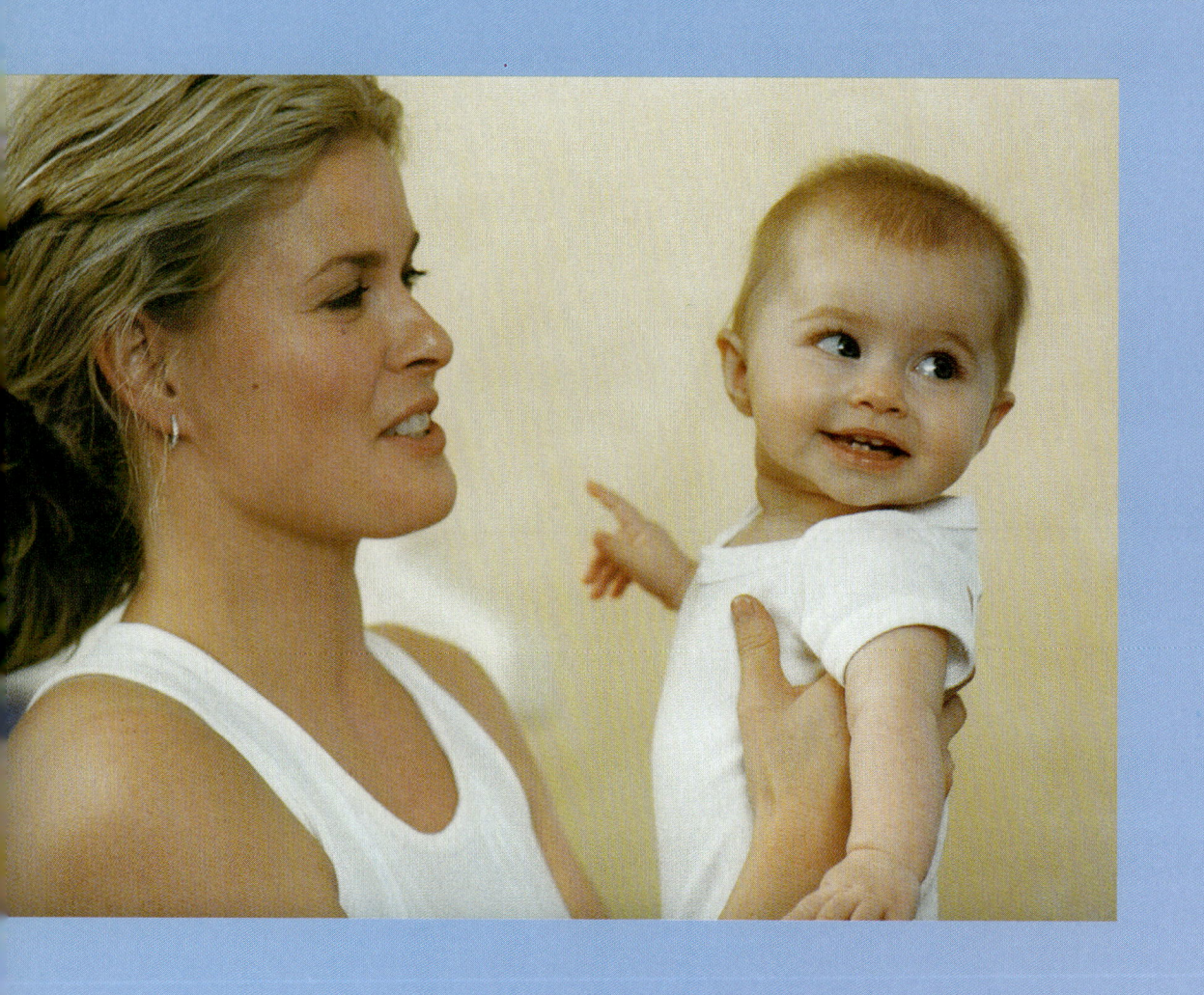

4

Boosting Your Body Image

Sometimes I feel as though I'm expected to look a certain way, especially because people are very intense about if you've lost the weight after you've given birth and how fast you've done it. That's really hard because the last thing you feel like doing when you're a new mother is being critiqued on the way you look. I've heard of people who look exactly the same as they did before they were pregnant within days of giving birth, but I don't know any of them. I mean, did those women have a plastic surgeon in the delivery room, performing liposuction while they pushed?

Exercise and proper diet are obviously the practical solutions for getting back into shape, and we'll deal in depth with those elements in upcoming chapters. But there are things you can do to make yourself feel better, even in the first six weeks after you've given birth, when you can't exercise at all (not like you'll feel like it!). Remember this: *It's natural to gain weight when you're pregnant. And it's natural to lose it again.*

Working in an industry in which one's weight is ridiculously important, I've had to deal with even my own agency telling me to lose a few pounds—just from looking at me. As if I might have missed it. If you are at all in tune with your body, you *know* when you've gained weight—your clothes don't fit as well, you feel different. You do not need to hammer the point home that you're heavier than usual by getting on a scale. Plus, it can become an obsessive activity, watching yourself gain or lose a pound. Your body has just done something absolutely amazing, and you have to give it credit. Your body knows what it's doing!

The period after giving birth is absolutely the wrong time to begin cutting back on what you're eating or to put yourself in a position where you're going to be feeling hungry. (I can't stand the word *diet* when referring to watching what you eat, and I promise, it won't be used once in this book.) Your body needs its strength. It needs to recover from nine months of pregnancy and labor, and if you're breast-feeding it also needs to provide nutrients for your baby.

Of course, that's all well and good, but the point is, your body isn't about to look the way it did before you got pregnant—at least not right away. So what can you do to feel better about yourself? A simple way is to forget about whether you're losing a pound here or a pound there. If your jeans feel looser at some point, great, but the actual number on the scale is irrelevant.

Another commandment to follow when it comes to liking your body again is this: *the mirror is not your friend.* For at least six weeks, avoid 'em. I'm not talking about that moment in the morning when you're brushing your teeth or when you're standing in front of a mirror before you go out making sure your shirt is tucked in. What I mean is, for the next

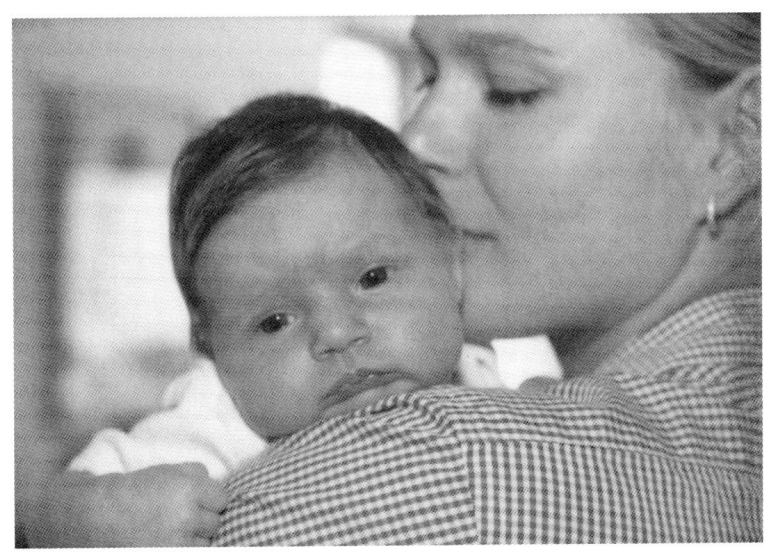

Spend your time loving your baby instead of looking at yourself in the mirror.

six weeks, tell yourself you are not allowed to obsess over your mirror image. No amount of staring at yourself while you're sucking in your stomach is going to change the fact that you've just had a baby and your belly is going to be bloated for a bit.

After my two deliveries, my stomach was like a doughy marshmallow, which made me really self-conscious. I would try to sneak into bed with my husband with a bathrobe on. But you have to think of yourself as something amazing that just gave birth to a baby, and celebrate your body—as nuts as that may sound.

There were days when I felt just awful, when I thought, "Who is this person? I'm never going to look the same again." Remind yourself that there are going to be days when you're going to feel amazing. And whatever you do, don't panic. It takes time to get back into shape, and after only a month or so, you're not going to be there.

Boosting Your Body Image

Also, never, ever forget the obvious: You're the one who notices, and you're the one who knows your body. I promise, no one else is looking at you thinking the mean things about you that you're thinking about yourself.

Here's another commandment to remember: *your prepregnancy clothes are none of your business.* There they hang, the first couple of months after you give birth, torturing you every single time you open your closet. Don't pay any attention to them. I was desperate to get out of my pregnancy clothes, but nothing is worse for your self-esteem than seeing if *just maybe* your favorite pair of jeans will fit. Trust me, they won't.

Soon enough, we're going to get you back into fighting shape with exercise and careful eating (you'll be satisfied, promise), but for the first six weeks, forget about it. Feeling tight clothes around your body is just going to make you feel worse, so improvise as much as you can.

To remind yourself that you're on your way to recovery, buy yourself a beautiful scarf, a pair of earrings, or a shirt that will fit you now and later. Splurge on a pair of shoes you've been craving or a luxurious sweater. I'm also an underwear fanatic, and I found that buying a lovely bra and underwear set can do a huge amount in terms of making me feel better about myself. There's no better time to celebrate your breasts (and remember, most men only look at breasts anyway, so don't sweat the size of your waist).

Two weeks after I gave birth to Hannah, my husband and I had to go to this extremely fancy wedding in Sweden, and I was completely stuck. I wasn't feeling even remotely attractive, and I didn't want to spend money on something I wouldn't wear again. I went to the department store and tried on a dress that looked OK from the front, but when I looked at it from the back I thought, "Oh, man, what's going on here?"

I managed to borrow a friend's dress with an empire-waist (meaning it had absolutely no waist) and plenty of room for my breast-feeding cleavage, but control-top panty hose are what helped the most. It's also helpful to occasionally wear a girdle under your clothes, just to remind yourself how you looked before and what you're going to look like again really soon. We *will* be getting you back into your old clothes, and in just a matter of months.

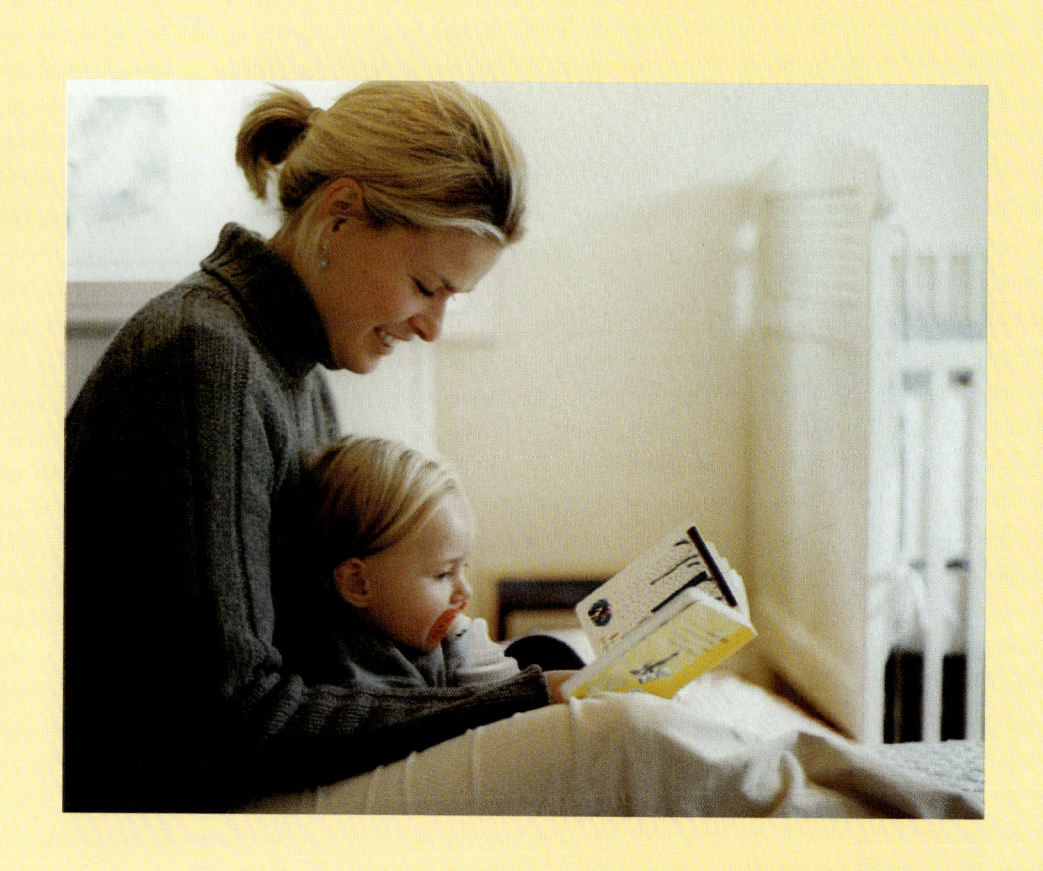

5

If You Decide to Breast-Feed

In part because of my work with UNICEF, I'm a big proponent of breast-feeding. Breast-feeding is a wonderful way to establish a physical bond with your baby, but there are many health benefits as well. For instance, you can greatly boost your baby's immune system, and studies have shown that the health benefits can last well after you stop breast-feeding. UNICEF studies have even shown that babies who have been breast-fed score higher on IQ tests when they're in grade school. (It's also extremely practical, especially when traveling. No matter where you find yourself, the kitchen's always open!)

But let me tell you—none of those statistics helped me when I ran into breast-feeding trouble with my second child. It had been so easy with Julia that it didn't occur to me to do the obvious: *get the number of a hot line or a lactation expert before you leave the hospital!* Right after I had Hannah, my breasts got terribly engorged because she was so sleepy she

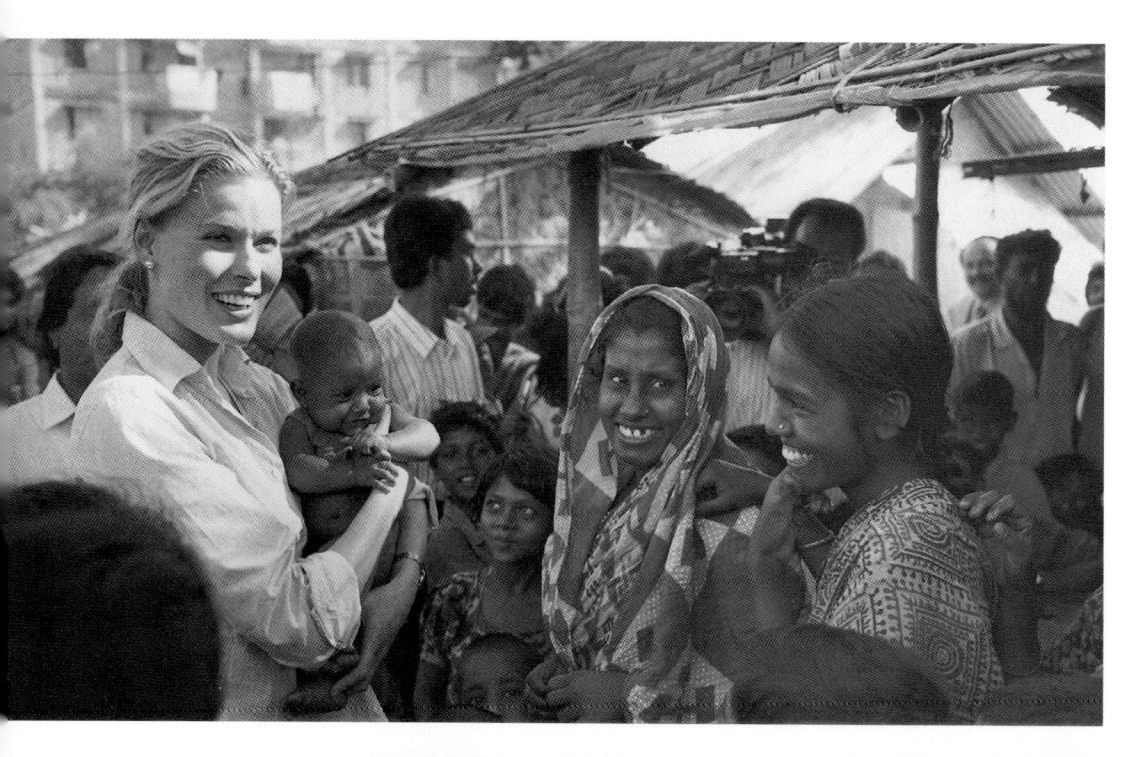

In my work with
UNICEF I learned
a great deal about
the value of
breast-feeding.

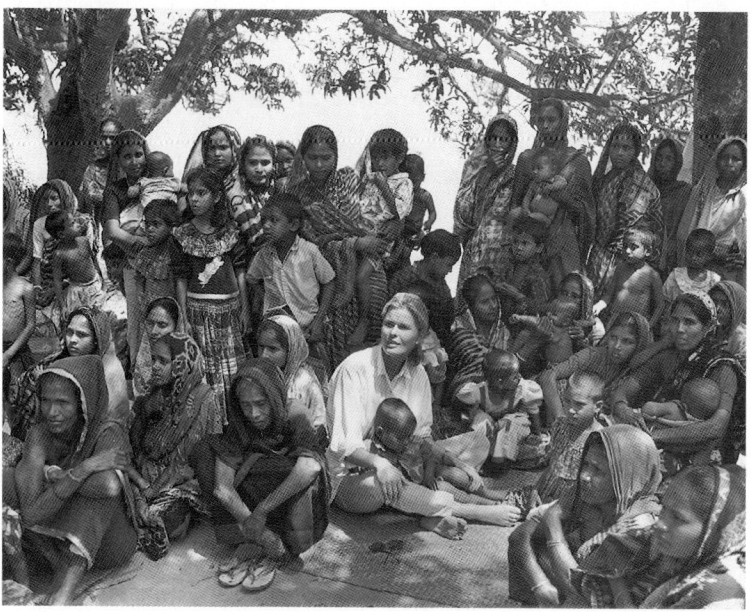

didn't want to eat. My fever went up over 104 degrees, and, because it was Memorial Day weekend, there was no one to tell me what to do.

It turned out to be as simple as getting the breast milk out by pumping—and wrapping a bag of frozen peas around my breasts to numb the pain—but I didn't know this in time to prevent myself from getting really ill.

Before you leave the hospital, get a number of a twenty-four-hour hot line. And if you're having trouble breast-feeding at first, remember, it's not your fault. Sometimes it's just tricky. If you can, stick with it. If you can't or decide you don't want to, that's fine. It's your decision and you shouldn't feel bullied one way or the other.

That said, Americans aren't necessarily receptive to breast-feeding mothers. If you can, ignore what you think people are thinking, because often they're not. One day I had to breast-feed in the supermarket, and I sat down in the aisle on top of some paper towels to do it. Much to my surprise, far from getting dirty looks, people came up and said, "That was really beautiful." (It's amazing how fast your definition of what's beautiful changes once you have kids!)

Obviously it's best to breast-feed at home. It's quieter, and you'll both be more relaxed, which means less indigestion. (Plus, no one will be coming up to you saying, "Our specials today are . . ." I've had a couple of spraying-milk incidents over that one when the baby suddenly got distracted and looked up instead of staying latched on.) In addition, if your baby is being fussy and you know that he or she is hungry, it can be helpful just to snuggle for a bit before breast-feeding. If you're bottle-feeding, you should also try cuddling first or lying down while you feed so that you have maximum physical contact.

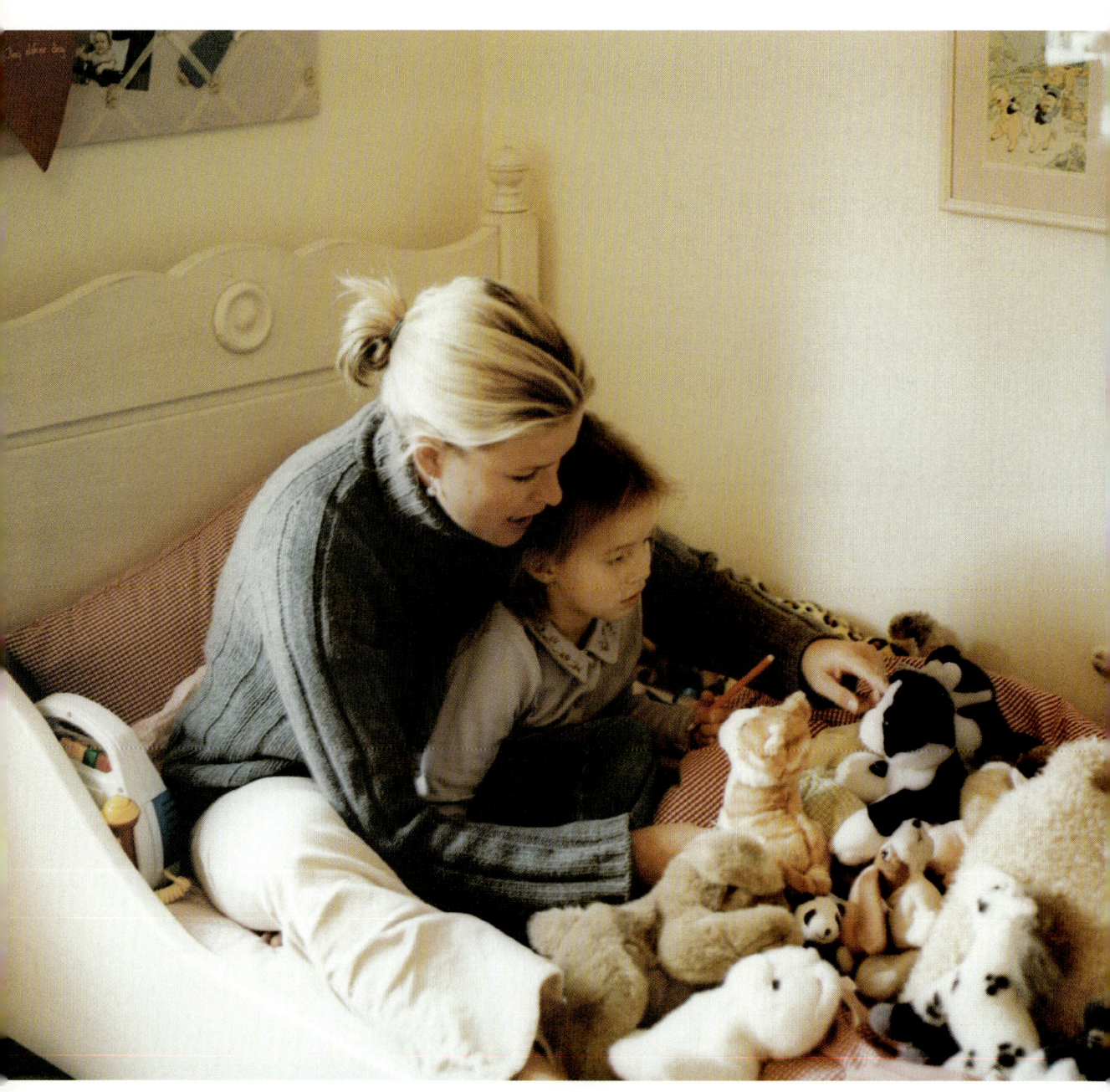

Whether or not you choose to breast-feed, lots of cuddling and close contact with your children is important, now and as they grow older.

Allow yourself a few weeks to find positions that work best for you and your baby, whether you use pillows or lie down, for example. I had found with Julia that lying down was the most comfortable for both of us, but Hannah didn't like lying down, so I had to reteach myself how to feed her. You'll know when you've figured it out because the baby will latch on more easily. I promise, if you can stick with breast-feeding, it will become second nature, but in the beginning it is normal for it to feel weird—it's not like either of you have ever done this before.

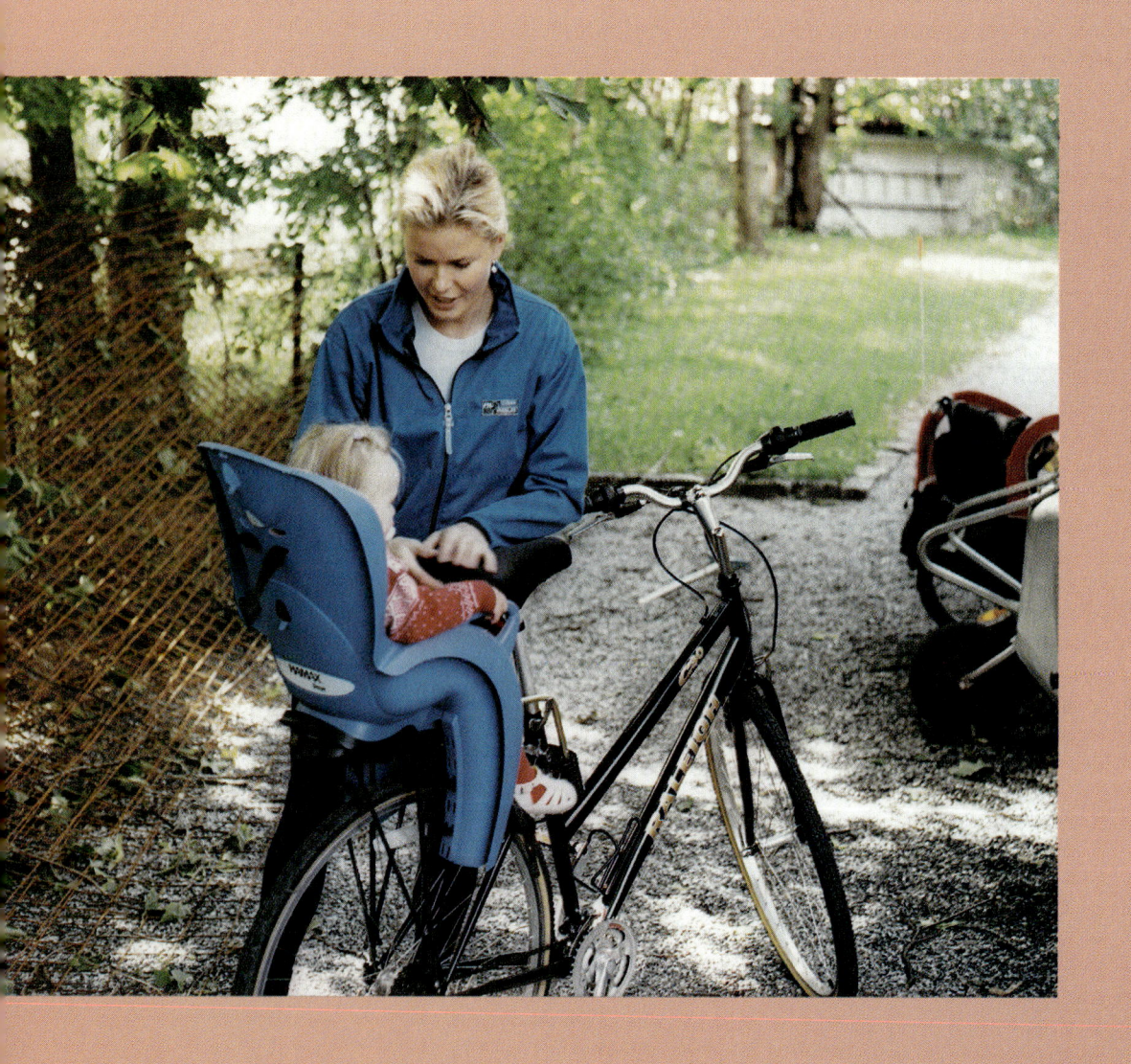

PART TWO

Exercise for Life

How to get in the right frame of mind and make the most of whatever time you have

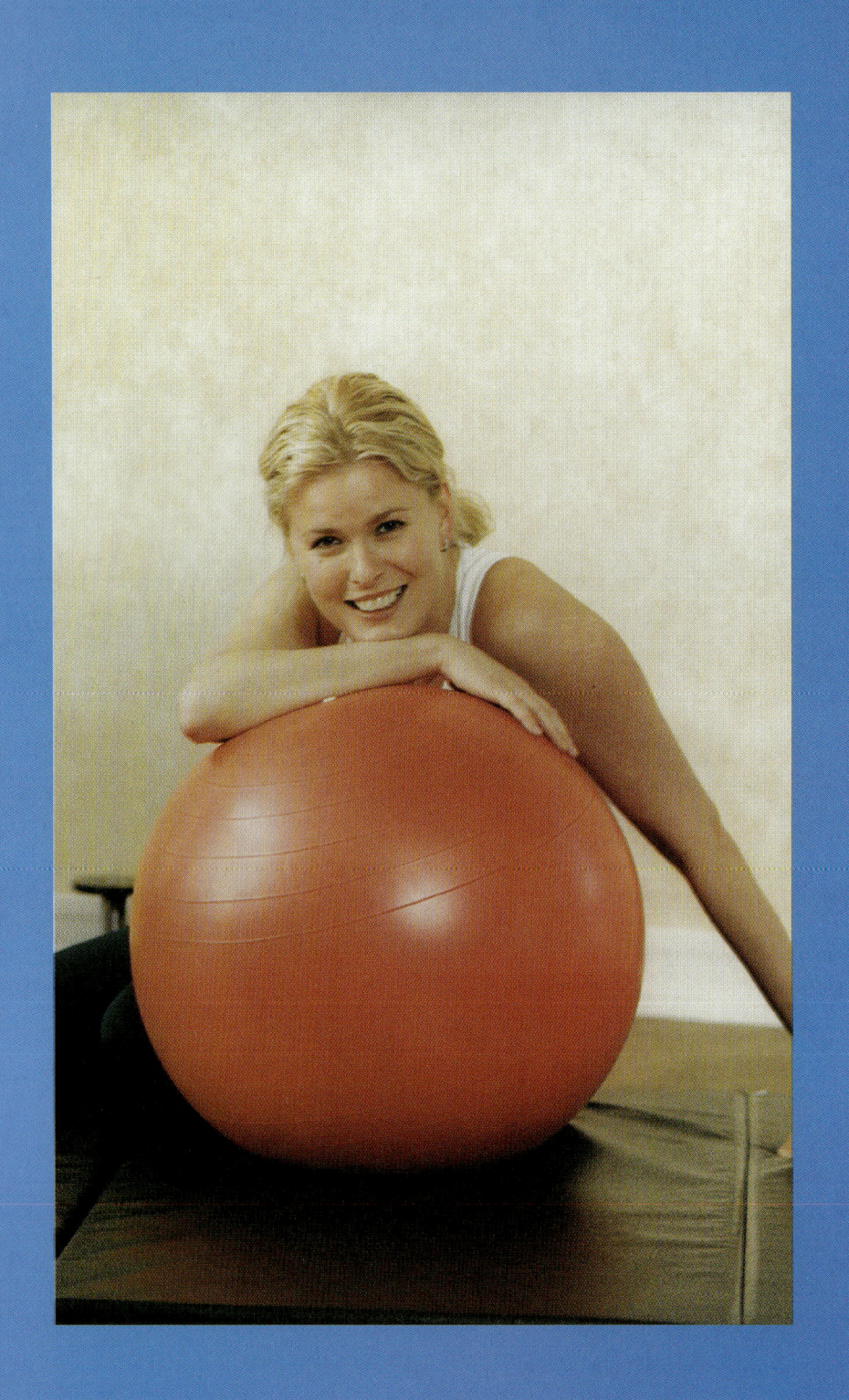

6

Find Your Motivation

Right before I gave birth to my first daughter, my husband and I had moved back to Norway for a few months. It was the dead of winter, and in Norway the sun shines for only a couple of hours a day during the coldest months. So needless to say, there I was, alone in a rented apartment, content to do nothing but eat and watch my growing belly.

The problem was that after I gave birth to Julia, I was still content to do nothing but eat and watch my gorgeous daughter. Plus, I was having wild cravings: chocolate, cake, cookies, ice cream, anything. I even had stashes of chocolate that I would hide from my husband—totally bonkers behavior.

Five months after I gave birth, I was still at least twenty pounds overweight. It was strange for me that none of my clothes fit, but I was happily settling into motherhood, and I didn't plan on going back to work immediately, so I wasn't concerned.

The second time was much harder. I had decided that I wanted to go back to work within a few months of having Hannah. Unfortunately, I literally *can't* work if I'm carrying any extra weight, so I asked for help.

I called Sean Kelleher, the personal trainer who had whipped my butt into shape for the *Sports Illustrated* cover, and he said, "Don't worry about it. Just show up." And since we'll take you through all of our steps, that's all you have to do too. But first, you have to get your mind and attitude ready to roll. Ready, set, let's go!

The first thing you need to figure out—and make sure to write it down when you do—is what your goal is going to be. Remembering why you're doing what you're doing is what guarantees your success.

For me, I focused on going back to work, which meant getting back into shape, unless I was going to be doing voice-overs. So I would remind myself that in order to do a commercial I really wanted to do, I had to tone up.

Pick something that's important for you, and hold it out there. Maybe you have a family member's wedding coming up, and wouldn't it be great to show off how fabulous you look? Or maybe you have a business presentation, or a vacation where you're going to want to be in a bathing suit. Write down what that event is and put it somewhere to encourage yourself.

As you know, being a new mother means often feeling out of control. Your whole life suddenly seems to belong to someone else! The time you carve out for exercise, even if you can only find ten minutes sometimes, is a present to yourself. You're doing something nice for your body and for your mind. At times a rush of endorphins and a burst of sweat can do more for your sense of well-being than eight hours of sleep— and there's little chance you'll be getting a chance to do that soon!

Equally important is that the time you take to exercise is time completely by yourself, with your own thoughts. (That's why I skip the headset and run in silence, unless I'm really

> **Motivation Tips**
>
> - **Make your goal realistic.** Aiming too high will just make you feel like you're failing. For instance, this isn't the time to decide you want to weigh what you weighed in high school. Once you get back to fitting into the clothes you wore just before you got pregnant, you can reevaluate your goals.
>
> - **Take it one step at a time.** In my closet I have two different sizes for when I've gained or lost a little weight. When you're thinking about which dress you want to fit into, pick one of your larger-sized outfits. When that fits comfortably, then you can think about fitting into a smaller one.
>
> - **Think of exercise as a reward.** I know that may sound crazy. There are days when I'm so tired I feel as if I can't muster up the energy I need to even go for a walk around the block. But the reality is I always, always feel better for having exercised, and all of a sudden, even if it's short-lived, I'm not tired anymore.

tired. Then it's all about Madonna). Even better, it's time no one can begrudge you, and it's time you shouldn't feel guilty about being away from your baby. I promise, no matter how little time you put into it, getting in better shape will make you feel better about yourself, which in turn, will make you a better mother.

Exercise is also used to combat depression. At a time when you may be feeling a bit blue or even have more serious postpartum issues, exercise can really help. (If you are feeling seriously depressed, please see a mental health professional or your family doctor immediately.)

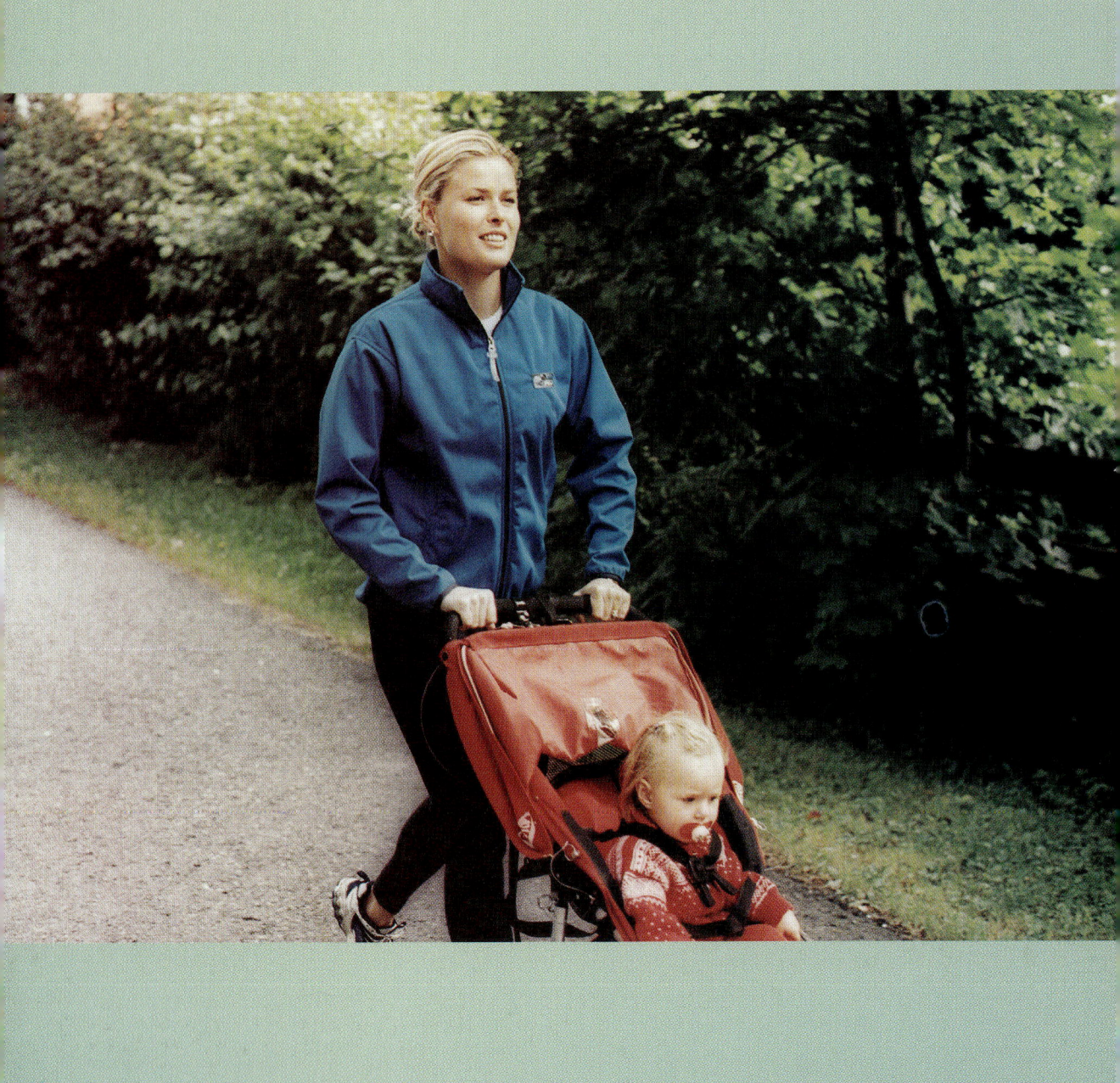

7

Choose an Activity You Like

I've always been someone who's happiest outdoors, so for me, going for a walk or a run in the park is the thing I like the most. Sometimes, though, when I'm really tired, I prefer to go to a Spinning or aerobics class at the gym, where the blasting music is a guarantee I'll stay awake. Plus, when a teacher's leading a class, you don't have to think about what you're doing. You just have to follow his or her lead.

Consider what it is you liked to do before you got pregnant. If you always enjoyed the social aspect of exercise, see if you can round up a couple of friends and catch up while you go for a run together. If you loved bike riding, head out to a trail and enjoy the fresh air. Whatever you choose, be sure to pick something that, when you think about going to do it, you don't want to crawl back under the covers and take a nap.

As you pick your activity, *be realistic about your limitations*. Like everything else in your life, workouts are going to be changed by having a new baby. First of all, you just aren't going to have the same time you had before—which is why we're going to concentrate on making the most of the time you do have. But you have to be careful about what you expect from yourself. Even if you were a marathon runner only months ago, your body has been going through so much and is completely discombobulated.

I didn't realize how tough it was going to be the first time around. Because I have always loved exercising and going for runs and because my pregnancy was pretty easy, I exercised up until my seventh month. (I didn't feel like it after that point, and I trusted my body that I should stop. I did the occasional yoga class but nothing aerobic.) So when I went out for my first run after having Julia, I thought, "How hard can this be?" After all, I'd been running regularly three months before, and I have been in pretty good aerobic shape my whole life.

Well, it was frigging impossible—and not just the first time out! The first run was so incredibly hard, I thought, "How can this be happening? I've been exercising my whole life!" I ran for about seven minutes and thought I was going to have a heart attack.

After having Hannah, I was better prepared. I knew that running wasn't going to stink just the first time. It would stink for a month. This is where it's really, really important not to get discouraged. You have to just keep at it. Tell yourself that the first month you can't expect *anything*. Maybe you'll be able to go from running for five minutes to running for ten minutes, but even that will be a major achievement!

I started out walking and moved up to running, very slowly. And then, instead of doing my usual six-mile run, I'd run for one mile. You have to just keep at it and remind yourself that every run is one run closer to feeling completely like yourself again. Remember: You didn't get out of shape while you were pregnant, *you got into pregnancy shape*. Your body has been working very hard over the last few months, so be kind to it!

You should also remember that it's an achievement in itself that you're even making time in your life to do something for yourself. The first time I made it back to the gym, I felt great that I'd made it there. And I felt proud that I was doing something that was heading me in the right direction. Your whole life has been taken over by a child, but this is for you.

OK—it's time to throw on your workout clothes (remember to wear two jog bras, especially if you're breast-feeding) and reclaim your body as your own!

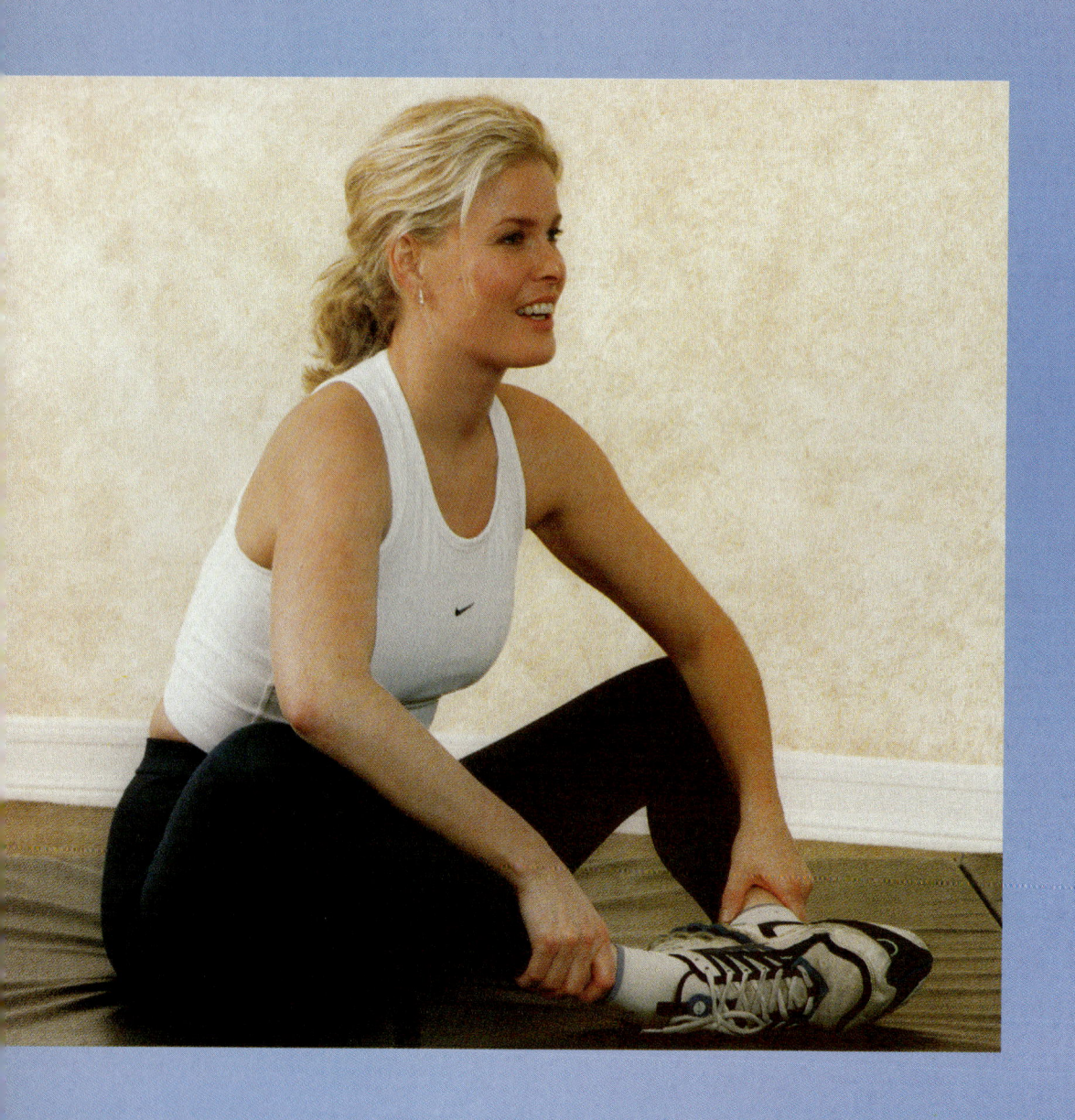

8

Time to Get Moving! Begin with Stretching

In an ideal world I would be going to the gym three times a week and doing a separate cardio workout two times a week. Of course, ideally there would be nine days in a week, so this would be possible. Remember that your goal is to get yourself moving as often as you can. If that means you have ten minutes to get your heart racing, that's still ten minutes of sweat and calorie burning!

This workout is designed so that you can be flexible and get a maximum workout in a minimum amount of time. That's why you won't see exercises that target one area of your body; your time will be much better spent using every muscle group. Believe me, you'll be amazed at how little time it takes to do three sets of lunges and pushups and how effective they can be!

Stretching is *crucial* to getting yourself back into shape and to feeling better. On days when I can't work out, I try to stretch for at least a few minutes—even if it's when I'm in the kitchen making dinner. It's been a long time since you've even been able to see your toes, let alone touch them, so start off easily.

After having a baby, you might notice that you're especially tight in certain muscle groups, such as your legs, which have been carrying around a lot of extra weight. Happily, you can stretch out your legs even while you're in bed or in the shower—this is one element of getting your body feeling better that you can do absolutely anywhere, and in only a few minutes.

Stretching is also an integral part of your workout. It helps prevent injury and alleviates muscle pain the day after exercising.

I used to stretch before I worked out, but with two children my schedule is so frantic that my warm-up now usually consists of rushing to the gym—believe me, by the time I've raced out the door and to my workout, I'm already sweating! But I always stretch out afterward. Here, are some crucial stretches you should incorporate into your workout—and, on nonworkout days, into your daily activities.

Sean helps me stretch my hamstrings, hips, lower back and glutes (or butt), obliques (or side muscles), inner thighs, and upper body. If you don't have someone to help you stretch, it's easy to do yourself—from your arms to your hips to your abs. Make sure to really focus on stretching your abs, because right after you've had a baby you'll tend to overwork that area in an effort to get the pooch out. By stretching your abdominals—arching up with your hands supporting you, as shown—you can avoid lactic buildup and cramping.

These basic stretches will reach all the important muscles you're going to use in the recommended workout; it's a good idea to do them before and after your workout. For each, bend until you feel a good stretch but not pain. Hold each for a few seconds.

Remember that you need to warm up your muscles before stretching. So either stretch after you've begun working out or run in place a bit first. Think of your muscle as a rubber band: if it's warm it will stretch pretty far, but a cold band will snap.

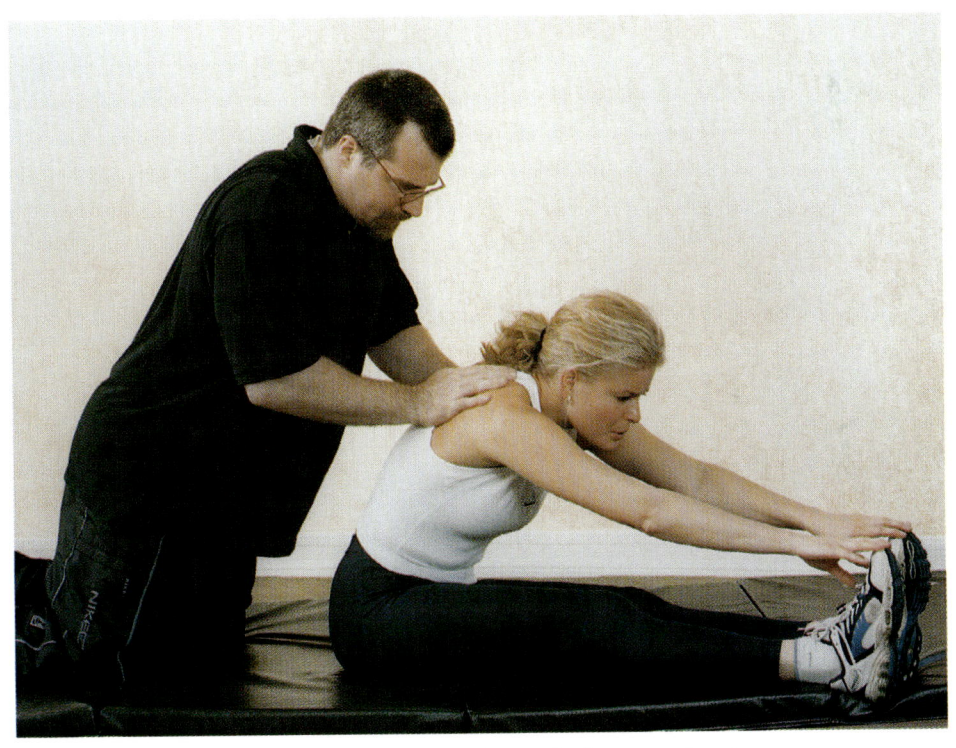

Hamstring stretches. To stretch your hamstrings—the long muscles at the back of your legs—sit on the floor with your legs straight in front of you. Grab your toes if you can, slowly bending toward them, and hold the stretch. If you can't grab your toes, wrap a towel around your foot and hold the ends of the towel.

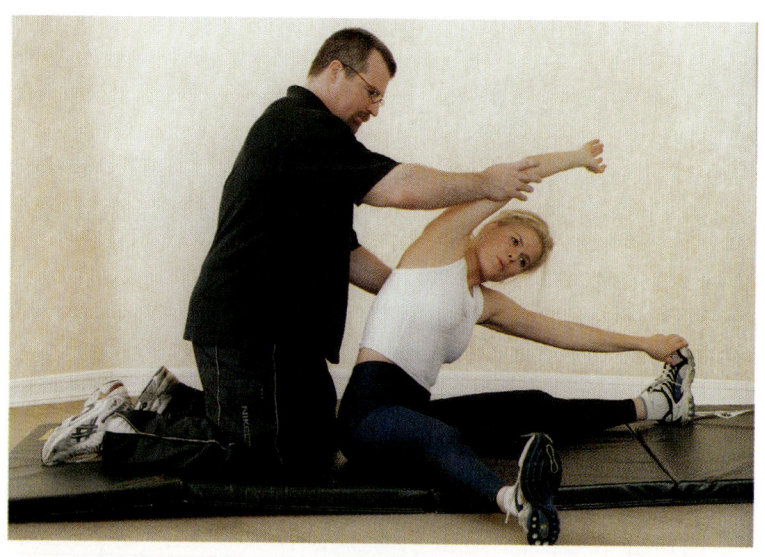

Next, spread your legs apart and grab your left toe with your left hand, or reach your arm out as far as you comfortably can. Reach your right arm over your head, keeping your right shoulder down, and stretch your body over your left leg. Feel the stretch in your side and your leg. Repeat on the other side.

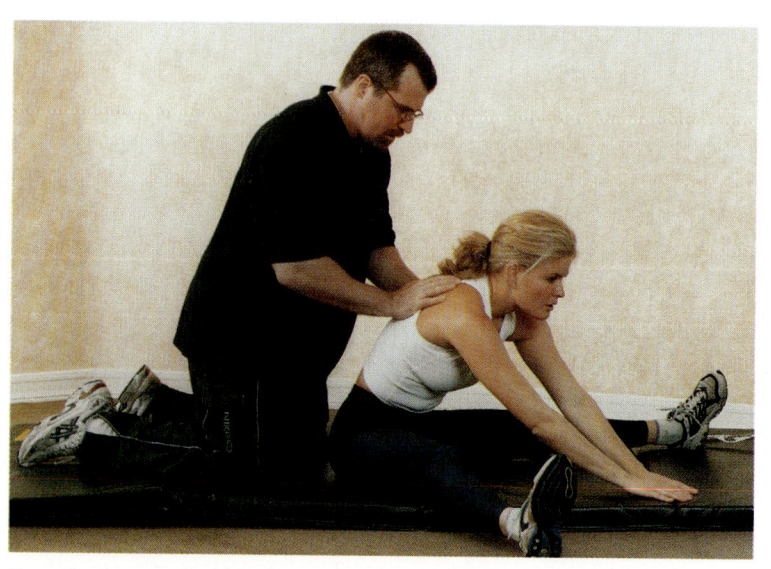

Face the front and reach your arms in front of you, then stretch your body forward and toward the floor, as far as you can comfortably go.

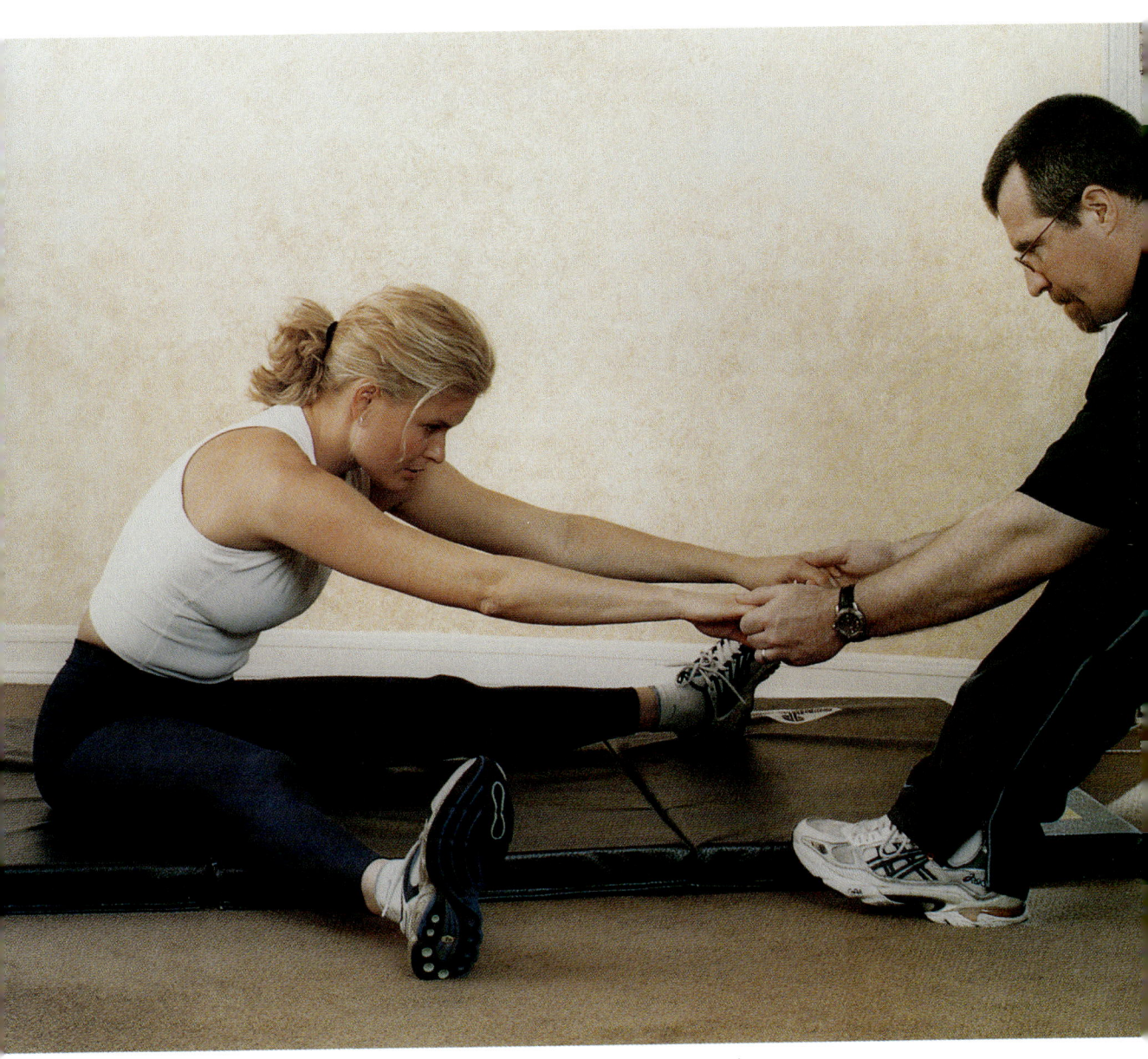

If you have a helper, have him or her pull your hands forward as you stretch.

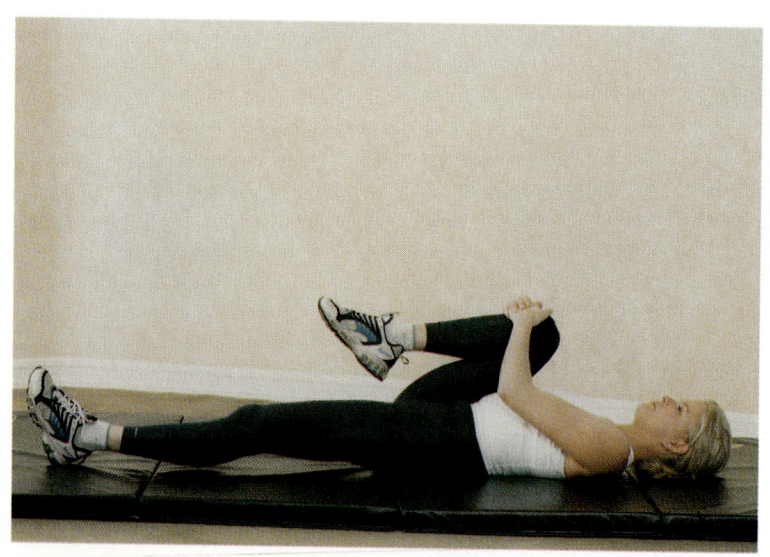

Hip stretches. Lie on your back with your right knee bent toward your chest. Keep your back straight and your butt on the floor. Grab your knee as shown.

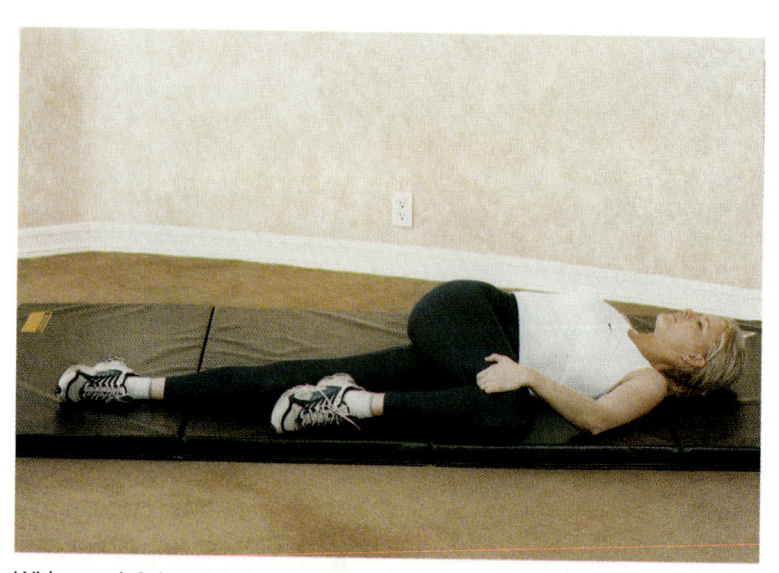

With your left hand, bring your knee over to your left side. If you can, touch your knee to the floor. Feel the stretch in your hips. Repeat on the other side.

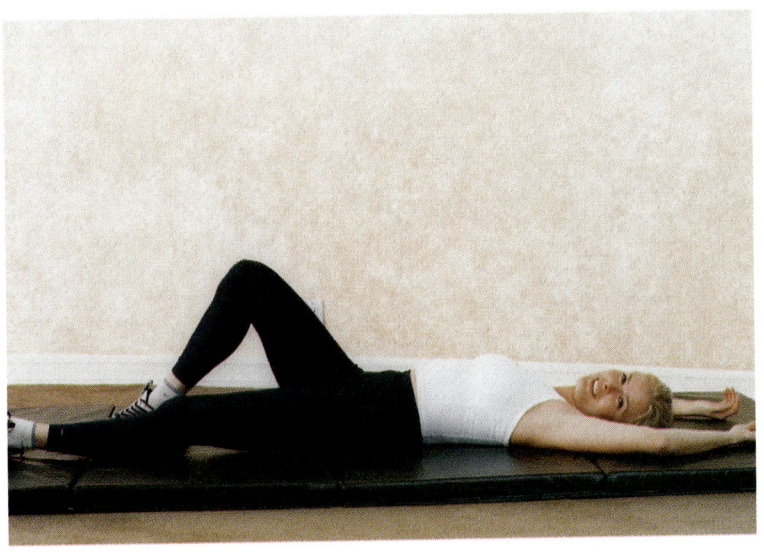

Lower back and glute stretches. Lie on your back and bend one knee up toward the ceiling.

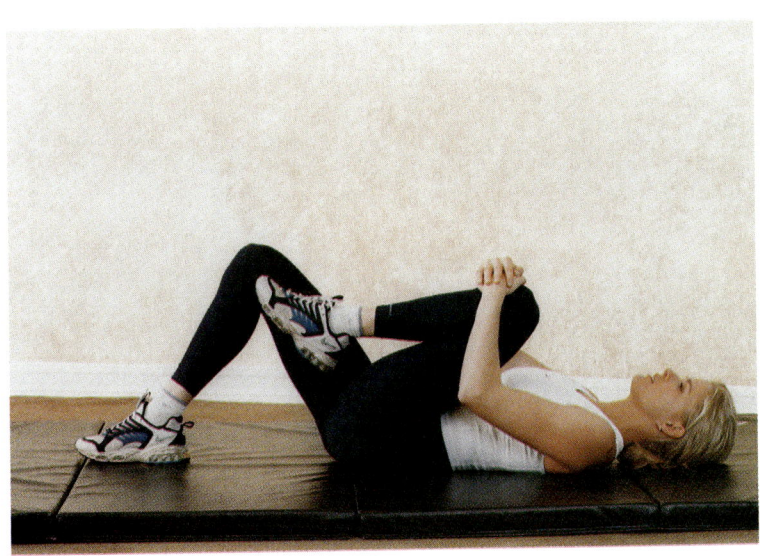

Bring the other knee toward your chest and feel the stretch in your lower back.

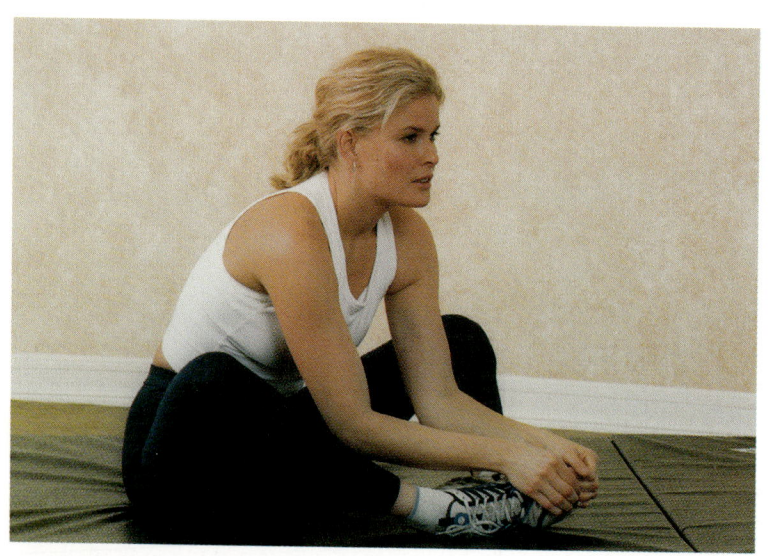

Inner thighs. For those inner thighs, sit with your knees bent and to the sides, the bottoms of your feet touching. Gradually push your knees closer to the floor.

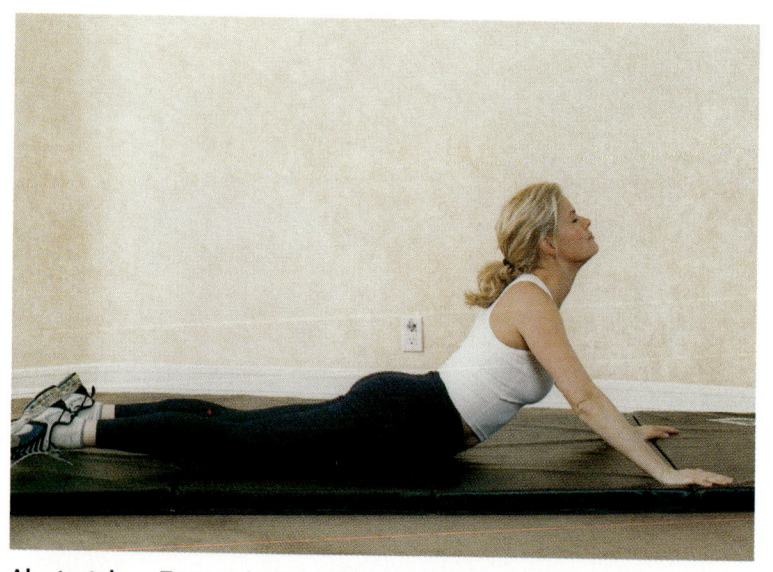

Ab stretches. To stretch those all-important abs, lie face down on the floor. Arch your back up, holding up your upper body with your hands, as shown.

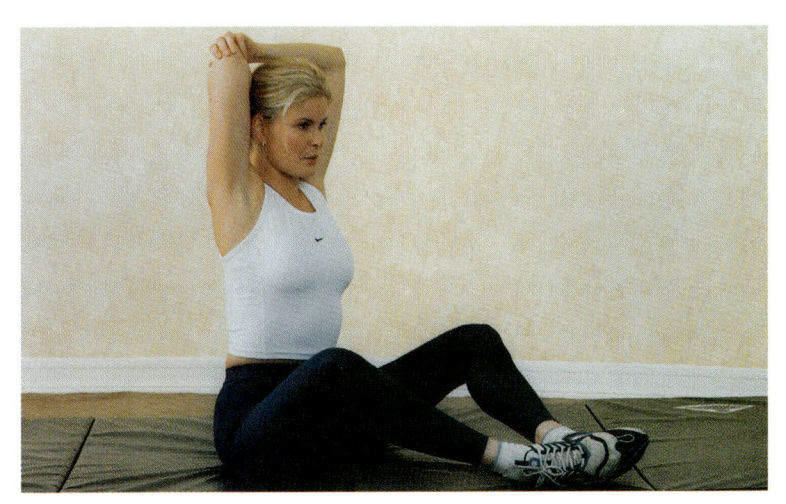

Arm stretches. For your arms, sit with your knees bent and out to the side, the bottoms of your feet touching. Raise your right arm straight up and then bend down your forearm so that your elbow is pointing toward the ceiling. Use your left hand to pull your elbow gently back. Repeat on the other side. If you find that your abs cramp during your exercise sets, do this stretch to help alleviate the cramps.

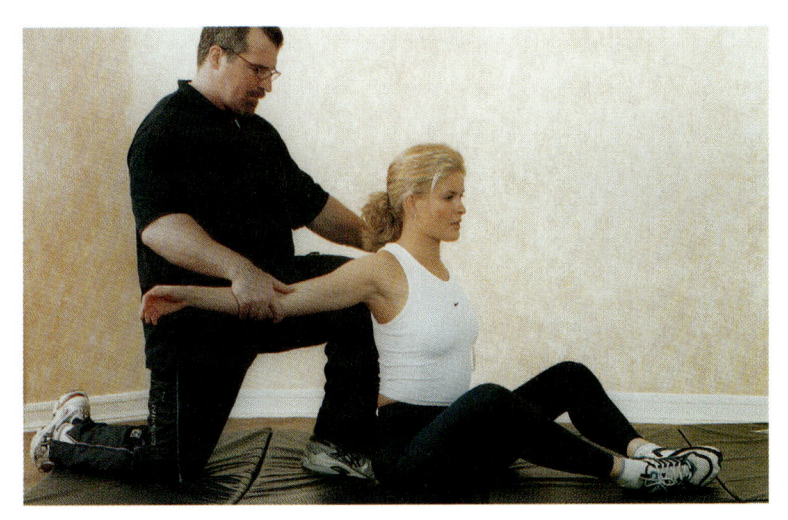

Upper body and chest. Remain seated and stretch both arms straight out to the sides at chest level. If you have a helper, have him or her gently pull your arms back. If you are on your own, stretch your arms back, keeping them at chest level.

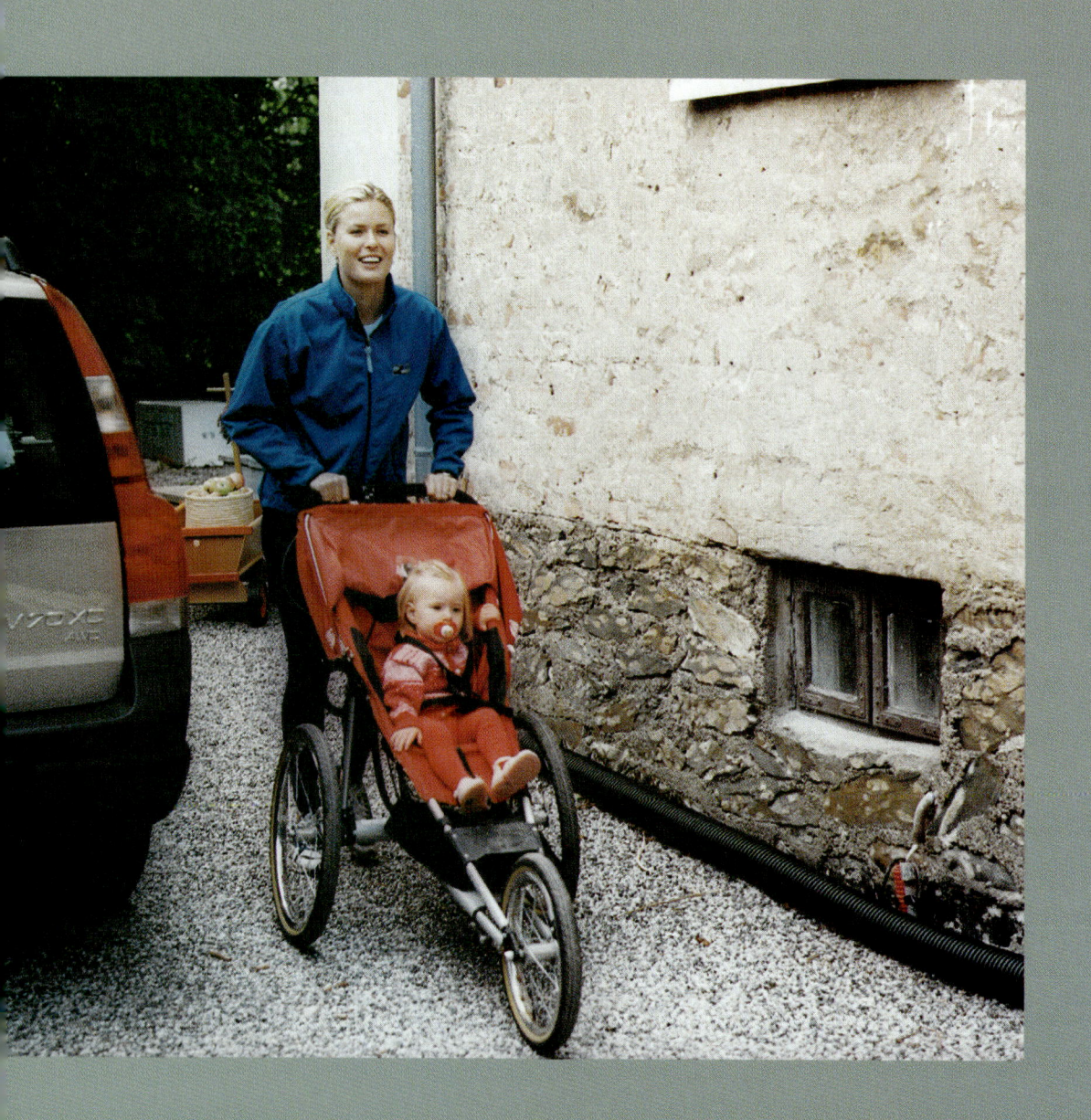

9

Cardio Work

If you have a minimum of time, you'll want to focus on cardio work. The strength training, which we'll get to in Chapter 10, is important in terms of getting stronger (obviously) and looking more toned, but right now the goal is to have more energy and lose that extra weight—and that means sweating.

Unfortunately, there's no shortcut. If you just watch what you're eating, you may lose a bit of the weight but probably not all—and it's still not healthy for you. The good news is that while there isn't a shortcut, *exercise works*. Period. If you start working out, you will see that your hard work pays off. And you'll see the results in a matter of weeks. (If you know your body well, you may see results in as little as a week, but don't expect anyone else to. If you don't see results as quickly as you were used to in your prebaby life, don't panic. It may take a bit longer than usual, but I promise it will happen.)

Remember, what's important is to do this for yourself and to feel good about yourself. This is a time in your life when

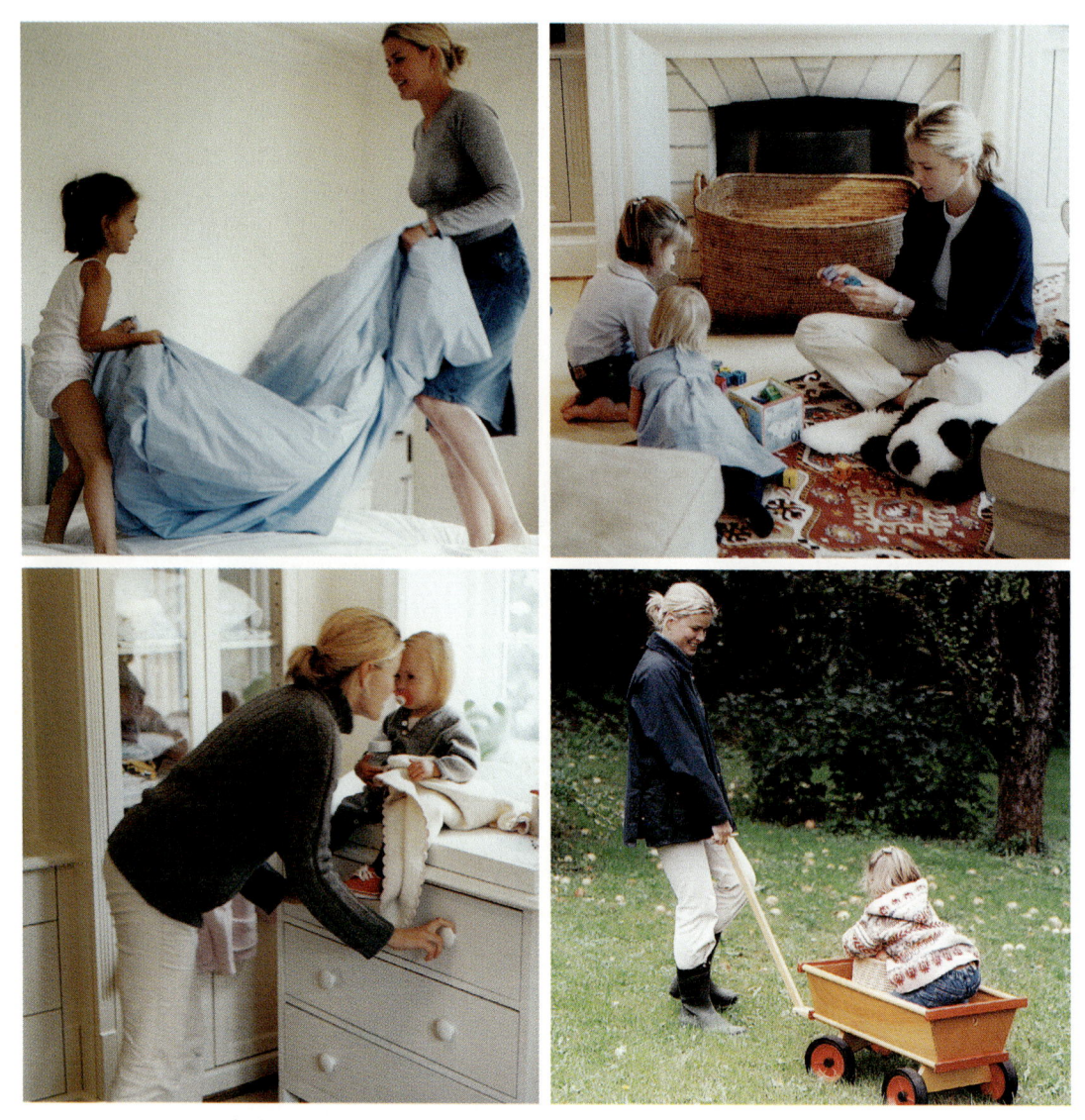

A little cardio work gives you more energy to enjoy your children.

it's important to make yourself proud and to get a lot of your self-esteem from inside yourself—it's not as if your baby is going to look up and say, "Wow, Mom—you're just amazing!" At least not yet. Working out can be a great and easy way to feel proud of yourself. In just twenty minutes, you will have done something you can feel good about for the rest of the day.

Even though doing an aerobic activity is probably the last thing you feel like doing right now when you're tired, I promise that an output of a little energy spent running or walking will give you hours of heightened energy in return. Plus, it's a great stress reliever, something I'm sure you could use a little of right about now!

That said, remember that the demands on your life are enormous, so don't get discouraged, even when you feel like you're back in shape and then you have a bad workout. I went for a run the other day and it was just impossible because I was so tired. You have to expect that. Sometimes your body just shuts down, and you should listen to it. I'm *not* saying that you can use a little tiredness as an excuse not to get moving—if you're not feeling slightly sweaty, you're not working hard enough. But if your body feels like it can't do it, it can't. Don't push it.

Your first workout should be ten to fifteen minutes. You can walk briskly or go for a slow run or alternate running and walking. Time yourself, and at the end of the time you've allotted yourself, *stop*, even if you're feeling great. It's important that you establish a sense of trust with your own mind and body, and if you've promised yourself that you're only going to go for fifteen minutes, then that's what you should do.

Cardio Work

Over the course of the next six weeks we are going to slowly increase the time and intensity of your workouts.

Your Aerobic Program

Be sure you have had a postpartum checkup with your doctor and have been cleared to exercise before beginning this program. As with any exercise program, check with your doctor if you have any health conditions that might be complicated by exercise.

Because your primary goal is likely to be fat burning, not long-distance training, this schedule will focus on that. If you're training for a marathon, you're going to work at 75 to 85 percent of your maximum heart rate. That's efficient aerobic training. But for fat burning, a lower heart rate is more efficient. The basic formula for the perfect fat-burning routine is to take 220 (your theoretical maximum heart rate) minus your age. Assuming you're 30, your maximum heart rate would be 190. For fat burning, you want to work at 65 percent of that, so multiply 190 by 0.65 and you get a target heart rate of 124 (hang in there—you just have to do this once, and we do allow a calculator!). Although 124 might seem too low, keeping to that rate is the most efficient way to burn fat.

Week One

For three days this week walk quickly for fifteen to twenty minutes each time. If that seems too easy, walk up stairs or hills to increase the intensity, or take your baby in a jogging stroller suitable for his or her age. Pushing that extra weight increases the workout!

Week Two
Add a fourth day of walking at the same level.

Week Three
Now we are going to increase the intensity. We're going to exercise four days for twenty to twenty-five minutes, doing any kind of aerobic activity, such as half walk /half jog, biking, or swimming. If you're biking, make sure to include a hill. This week you want to be sure to break a sweat.

Week Four
This week we want to increase the volume to twenty-five or thirty minutes but keep the same intensity. Remember: soreness is not an indication of your fitness level. You are introducing yourself to a new exercise, and soreness tells you that you haven't done this before. You can reduce the amount of muscle soreness you experience by stretching thoroughly and cooling down. The best piece of advice is that you work up to pain, never through it. The Olympics are not in your future here, so let's keep that in mind.

Week Five
Now it's time to increase the intensity again. You want to work at a higher level, with your heart rate between 65 and

75 percent of your aerobic zone for twenty-five of those twenty-five or thirty minutes. At this point you know you can do it, so skip the easing into it. You still need to warm up, but pick up the pace immediately, whether you're riding your bike, running, or swimming. Do this for four days.

Week Six

Time permitting, increase to five days a week, keeping the same intensity level.

Maintenance

After week six, find your own rhythm for your maintenance program. The above is goal oriented; once you obtain your goal, move into your maintenance program. Try to work out at least three times a week, even if it means shorter workouts.

Remember: body fat is a part of human nature, and it's important, especially for women who are childbearing. In fact, a certain amount of body fat is necessary in order to conceive at all. So keep your expectations realistic and healthy. We want to make you more comfortable with your body and in doing so make you healthier and stronger.

What Happens When You Get Off Track

While it's a good idea to use the schedule above as a guide, don't get upset if you find that you've gotten off the program occasionally. It's going to happen, and *that is not an excuse to abandon it.* Now that you have a baby, you're going to be forced to be more flexible, and this is a good place to start!

One trick that I use that's been immensely helpful is that I give myself five "passes" a month. That means that five times a month, when something comes up or the baby-sitter doesn't show up or I have a meeting, I can skip my workout that day. All right, so usually it's just that I have to sleep, I admit, but by giving myself the "passes" in advance, I don't beat myself up for having had to skip my cardio routine. The passes become a part of the routine, so it's not like I've fallen off the wagon.

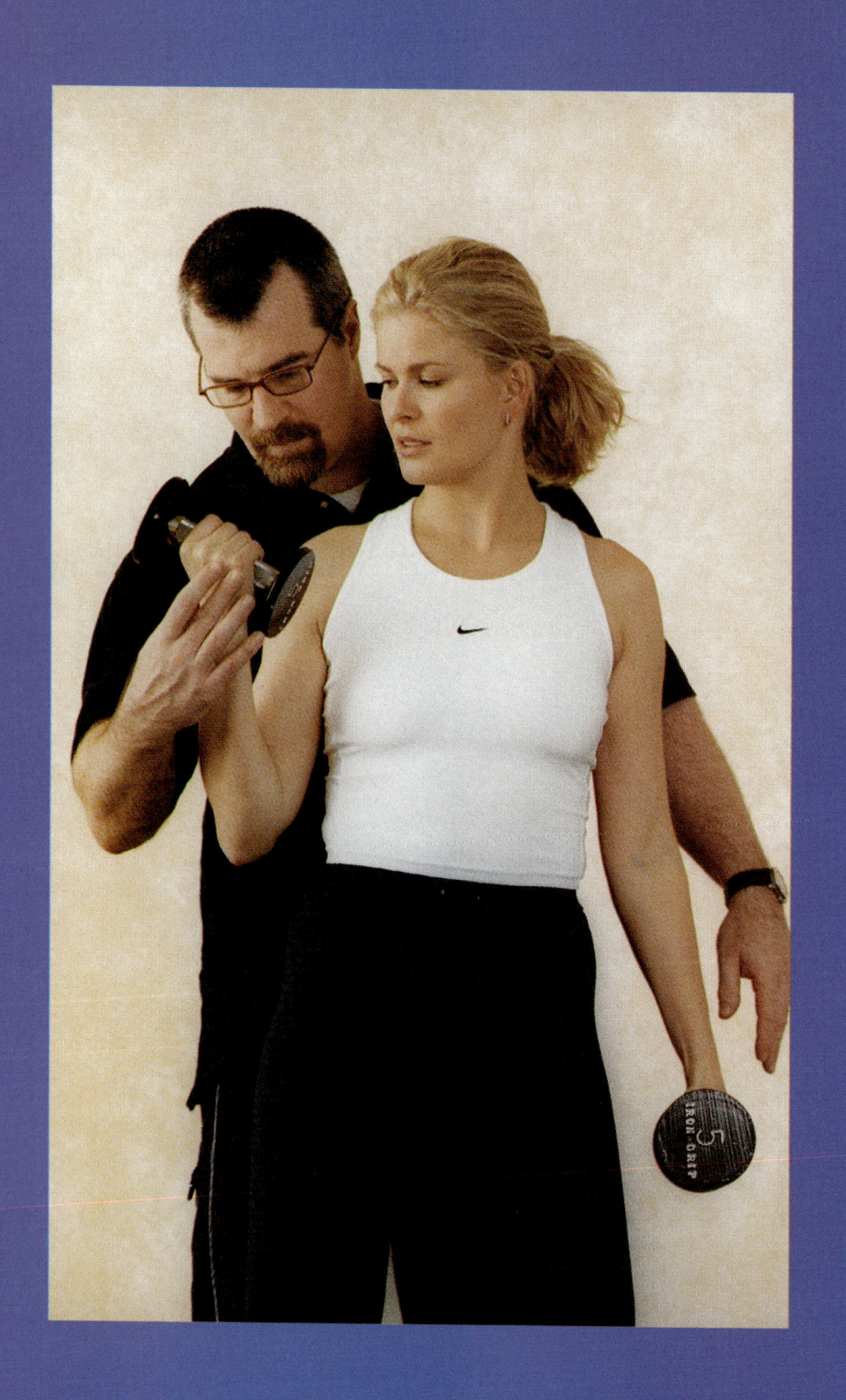

10

Strength Training

I never guessed that strength training would be so important after having a baby. Suddenly, there I was constantly picking up my babies, hauling diaper bags around, schlepping strollers—you have to be in good shape just to get you and your baby out the door!

My trainer, Sean Kelleher, has worked with me to get me into the best shape of my life—in less time than it's ever taken. Believe me, this guy does not mess around. That said, this workout is totally manageable; Sean completely understands that if he makes me too exhausted, that's not going to be a workout I can stick to, especially being a working mom. Unlike cardio work, which never gets easy for me, you can see a difference in workouts with strength training almost immediately. If you can do only five squats your first workout, it's very likely you will be able to do seven the next time.

Every routine that Sean's given me and that I am passing on to you is based on the principle that targeting smaller muscles is a waste of your time. Exercises should be based on multiple joint, or compound, movements, which means that you're using your largest muscle groups. Some videos from a few years ago had you doing little leg lifts here, little arm things there—that doesn't work. To get into shape, you have to work the big muscles, your glutes (or tush—it's hard to miss these days, isn't it?); your quadriceps, or thigh muscles; and your hamstrings.

Here's the deal: Even though strength training isn't officially a cardio activity, you still have to sweat. If you're not sweating, you're probably not working hard enough. These exercises are based on the idea of doing repetitions. As we get your body stronger, we will increase the repetitions; we're also going to cut down on the time between sets. So if you start out, as I'll show you below, doing five lunges followed by a rest followed by a couple of pushups, we're going to get you up to doing twelve of each, with no break in between.

The idea is to make the most of your limited time. I promise that even if you just do ten minutes of strength training a couple of times a week, you *will* see a difference. And think how great you'll feel when you can do ten pushups without collapsing!

In a perfect world you would have one day to work on a certain muscle group, say your arms, and then do your legs on another day. But who has that kind of time? This workout is going to get you working all of your muscles all of the time. The idea is that you work out your legs with something like squats, and then go right to arm exercises, which give your legs a chance to rest, while you're keeping your heart rate up and decreasing the time you spend standing around.

Before you do any of these exercises, make sure to take at least five minutes to warm up. I used to run to the gym, but now I'm always running late and carrying three bags, and that's my workout! (Please remember that while I usually go to a gym, all of these exercises can be done in your living room with your baby right there next to you.)

Again, don't push yourself so hard that you don't feel good—it's not healthy for your body, and you may not go back to the routine. The goal is to get your body back into training, which means that each workout is going to build off the workout before it. Push yourself too hard one day and you won't be recovered in time for the next workout. You want to take it slow and build your way up.

Sean's Quick Philosophy to the Perfect Workout

- **Use your full body.** No one has time to work out a different body part on different days. Do exercises that work more than one muscle group.

- **Work from bigger to smaller.** Start with large muscle groups (glutes, legs), and progress to small groups (arms).

- **Range of motion is crucial.** Each exercise should go through the entire range of motion. Don't cheat.

- **Build up your intensity.** You can increase intensity by adding weight, adding repetitions, or decreasing your resting time between sets.

- **There's no such thing as spot reduction.** You will tighten, strengthen, and tone through exercise, and you will burn calories, but losing weight is about eating better as well as exercising.

Strength Training

Here are the exercises. Remember: *the goal is to get in and get out.* Maybe there are people who have three hours to take classes and lounge in the whirlpool, but in your world, people don't live that way.

Strength Training Exercises

All standing exercises begin in this position:

1. Feet shoulder-width apart, slightly turned out for balance
2. Knees slightly bent to relieve pressure on your back
3. Back straight—pay attention to your spine's alignment
4. Head straight and looking straight in front of you to prevent neck tension

As I said, you always want to do your big muscle groups first, since those take the most energy. Therefore, you'll want to start with your legs. We're going to do exercises that require compound movements, which means more than one muscle group is working during the exercise. That way you can make the most of your limited time.

Squats

One of the best ways to work your legs is with squats—they're simple and killer. As you can see in the pictures, there are three

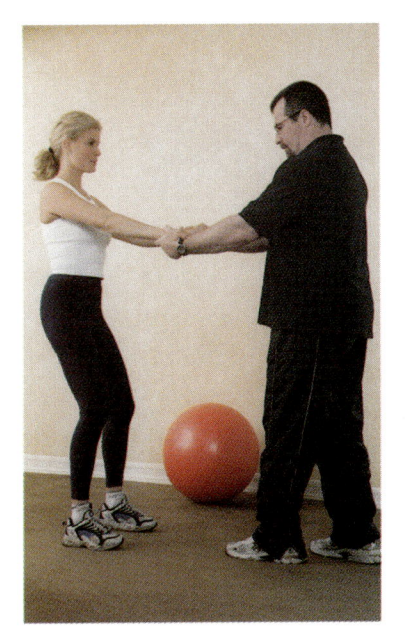

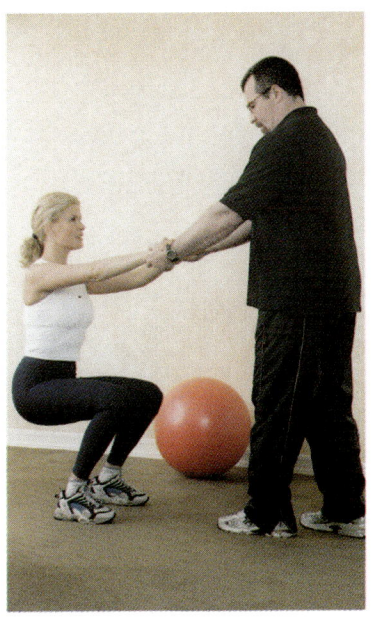

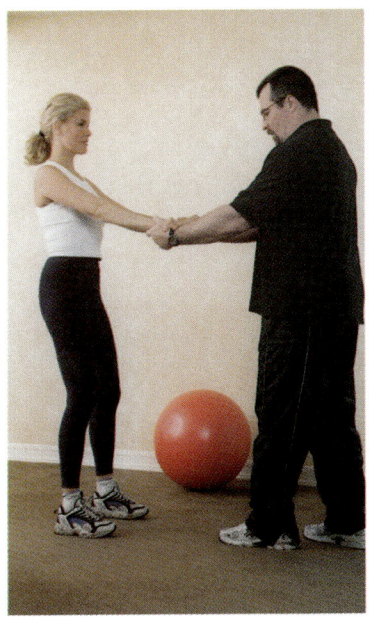

Squats. You can have a partner hold your hands for balance as Sean does for me here. Begin standing with your feet hip-distance apart and your back straight. Squat down to a 90-degree angle. Return to a standing position and repeat. Start with just a few, then build up over the next six weeks to three sets of fifteen or twenty reps. Do the movement slowly but fluidly.

Strength Training

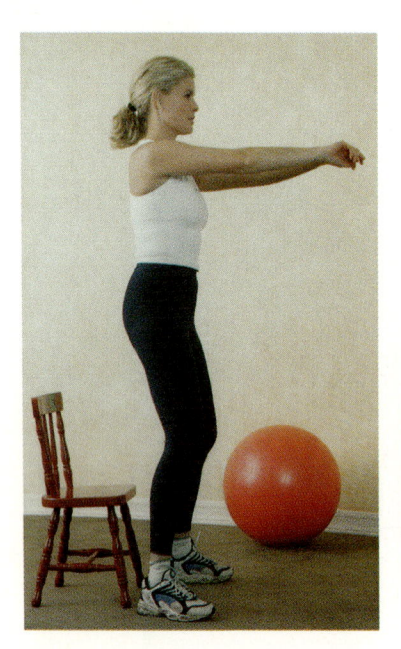

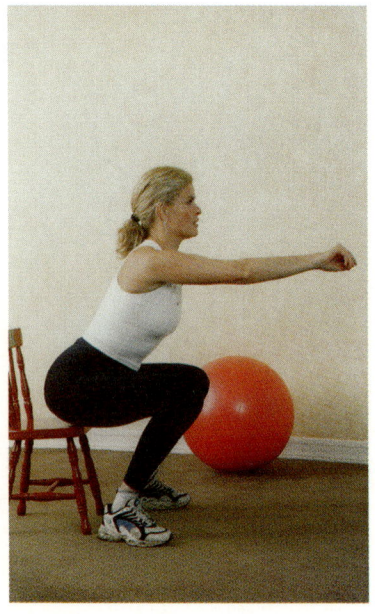

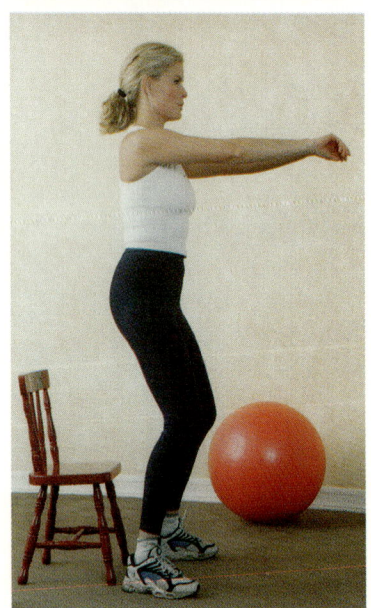

If you don't have a workout partner, you can use a chair, as shown, so that you don't fall on the floor. Squat down so that the backs of your thighs are parallel to the chair. Your butt should just touch the chair, but your weight should not rest on it. Do the squats as instructed on page 69.

70   EXERCISE FOR LIFE

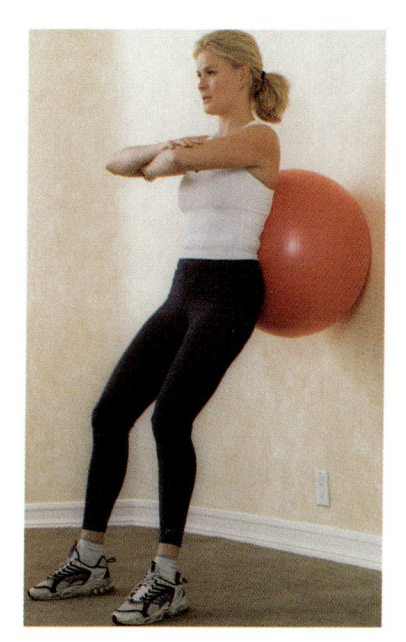

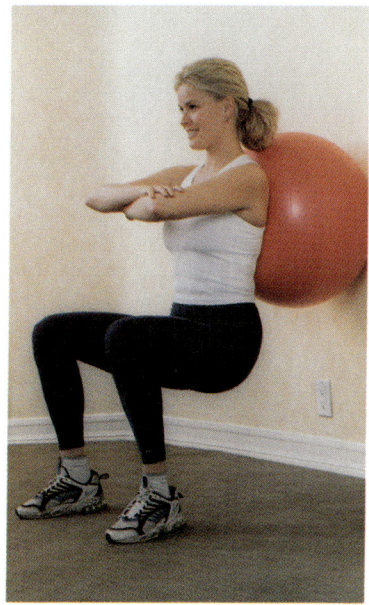

In another variation of the squat, you're going to use a ball—they're inexpensive, great for working out, and easy to store, so go pick one up at a sporting goods store. Rest your back against the ball and as you squat, come down to a 90-degree angle, with the ball sliding down the wall behind you. This works the same muscle as the chair squat, but is a bit more advanced and increases the intensity because you're adding balance, and the ball makes you keep your back totally straight, so you're really forced to use your glutes.

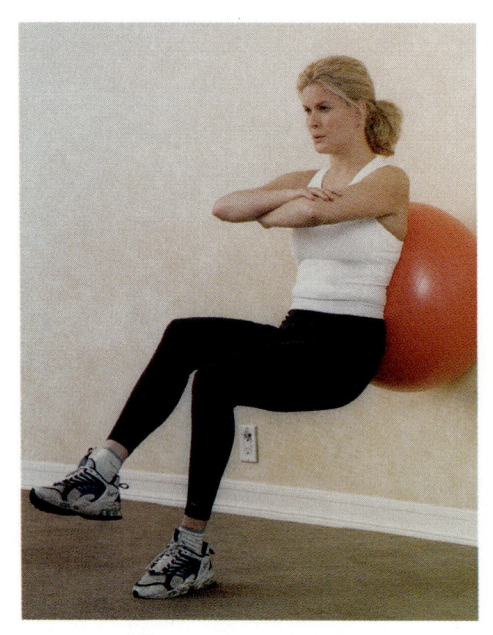

When you've nailed squatting with the ball, try lifting one leg at a time, so you can focus on a single leg. With this step you're introducing bilateral strength and balance.

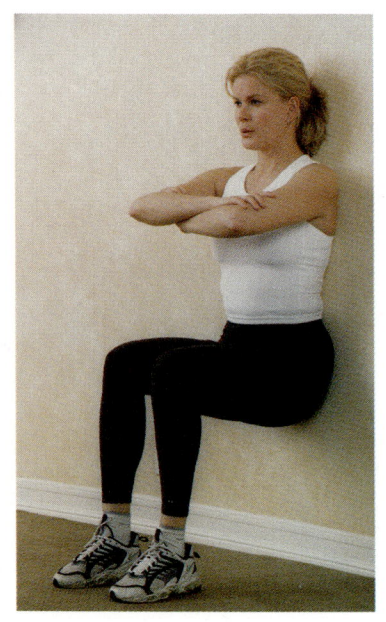

For the final variation, do what we call the wall sit. This is the easiest in terms of coordination but the hardest on your legs. Simply rest your back agains the wall with your legs at a 90-degree angle for forty-five seconds. Work up to ninety seconds.

variations. None of them needs to be done outside of your living room, but all allow you to increase intensity and strength.

Plies

A plie (pronounced PLEE-ay) is a knee bend with your legs turned out. They work your glutes and inner thighs—and man, do they work them.

Begin by standing with your feet flat on the ground and spaced wider than your shoulders, toes turned out. Now bend your knees so that they go over your feet, and lower yourself down until the backs of your thighs are parallel with the ground. The key to the plie is to keep your back straight and your weight in your heels. Your first instinct is to arch your back when you get low, but keep your abs tight and butt tucked in to avoid back injury. Really concentrate on those muscles and be aware of pushing with your glutes and inner thighs. It's not a bad idea to start against the wall so you can

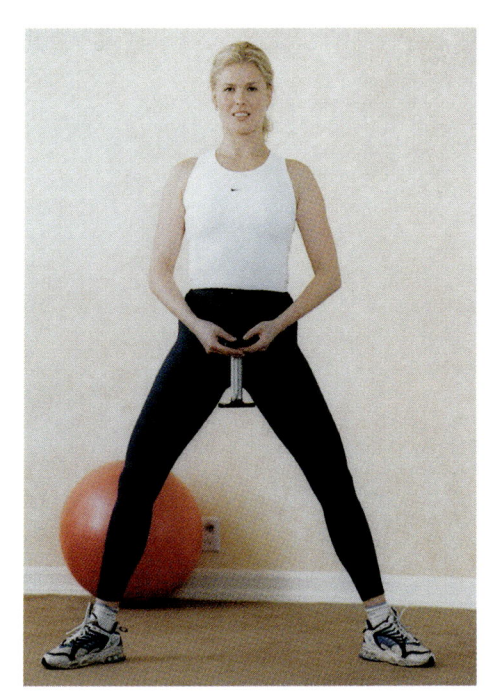

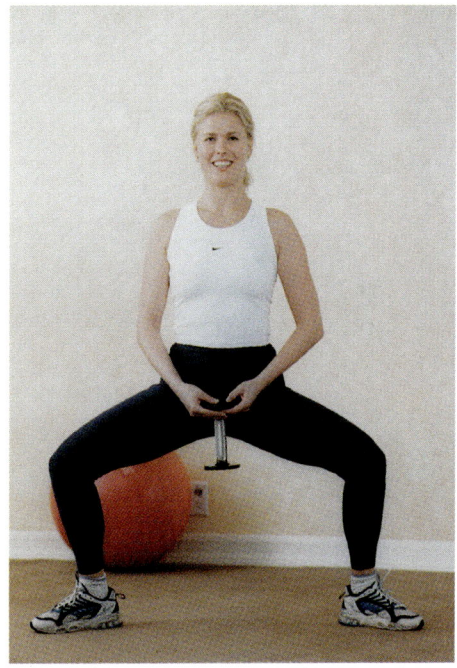

Plies. When you can do regular plies (week two or three), it's time to add a dumbbell, which you'll hold in your hands, just to add resistance.

Strength Training

feel what your back feels like when it's perfectly straight. Work up to three sets of ten to fifteen reps. After two or three weeks increase the intensity by adding weights. Aim for five pounds in each hand.

Lunges

This is another one that seems simple but where alignment is everything, both for maximum workout and to prevent knee

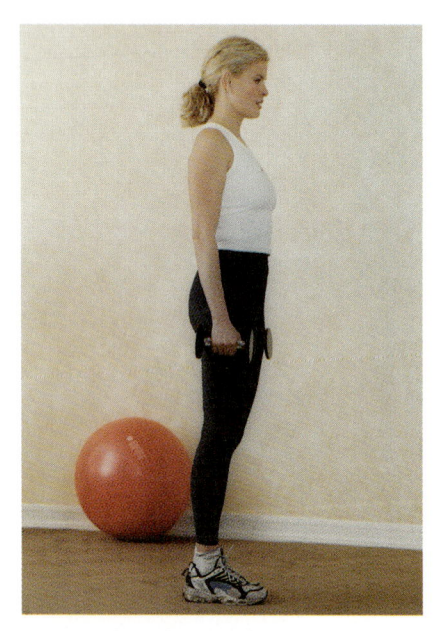

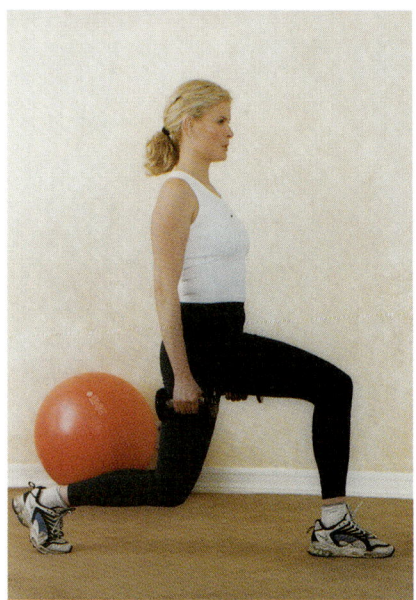

Lunges. Start by standing straight, feet hip-distance apart. Extend your right leg to the front, plant your foot, and transfer your weight to that leg, bending your right knee. *Be very careful that the front lunging knee is in a straight vertical line with the ankle, never with the knee extending beyond the ankle.* As always, keep your back straight by holding your lower abs tight and tucking in your butt.

injuries. As with all of the exercises, be sure to look straight ahead. Looking down can cause you to round your back.

There are two variations to the lunges: You can alternate legs, staying in one spot or you can do a walking lunge, for which you'll need more room. If you have the space, this latter variation is usually better because you don't shorten your stride as easily when you start to get tired. Work up to three sets of ten to fifteen lunges on each leg.

After two or three weeks increase the intensity by adding weights. Aim for five pounds in each hand.

Pushups

With pushups, we're moving on to your upper body. You may not feel like your upper body needs as much work as your lower body, but it's important to have a balanced workout, and it will make you look better in your clothes. Plus, picking up your baby day in and day out, you better have a strong upper body to avoid back injury and just feeling exhausted!

Dumbbell Press

The dumbbell press is going to work your shoulders and triceps. Range of motion is important here—when you raise your hands above your head, you want your elbows almost fully extended but not locked. Locking your elbows causes stress on your joints and rests the muscles that you want to work. You should start with two five-pound hand weights and gradually move to more weight.

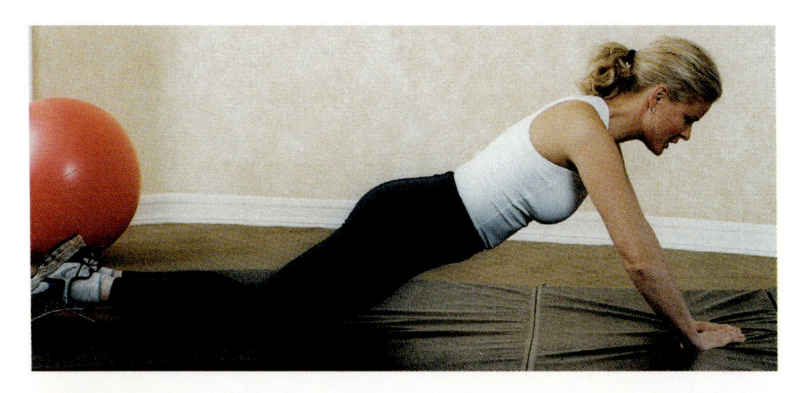

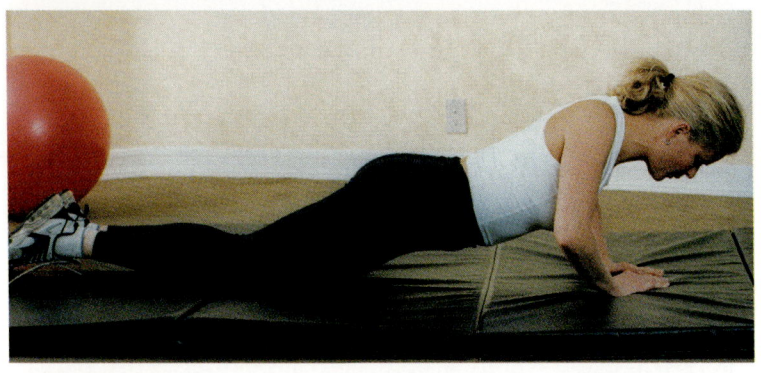

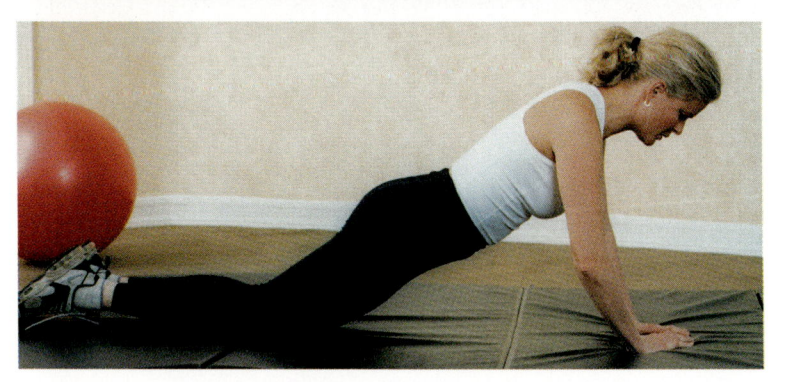

Pushups. Start doing pushups on your knees, lowering your upper body down on bent elbows, keeping your back absolutely straight. It looks easy, but again, doing it right will work out not only your pecs, shoulders, and triceps, but also your abs because they need to be tight to stabilize you. Start with three sets of eight to ten reps, and work up to fifteen.

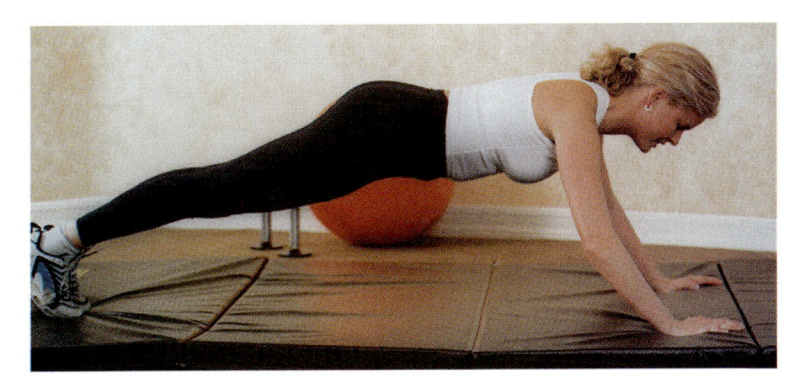

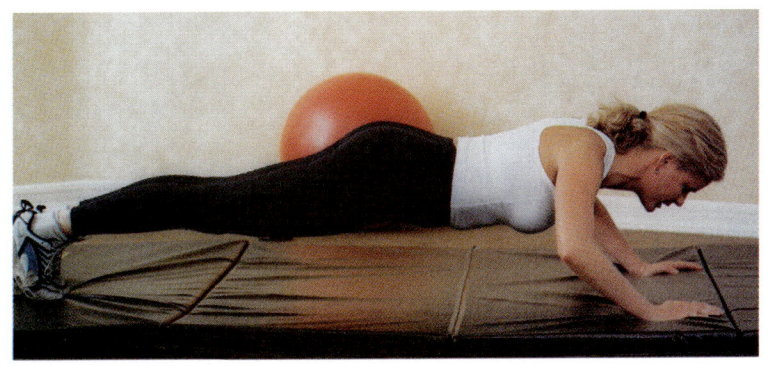

When you can do three sets of fifteen pushups with relative ease, begin to increase the intensity by moving from your knees to your feet—the traditional pushup.

Strength Training

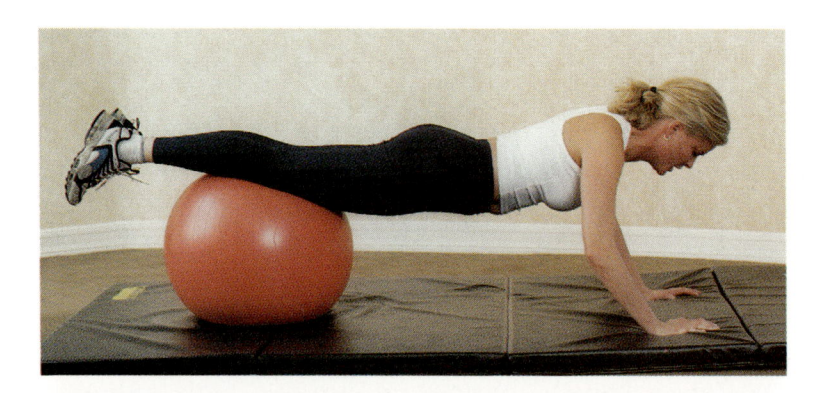

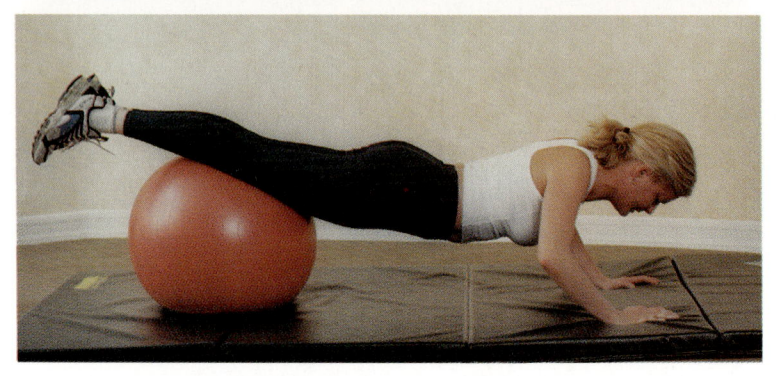

Then, if you're really feeling strong, go to pushups on the ball. The ball is really advanced and takes a lot of balance, so don't kill yourself trying this!

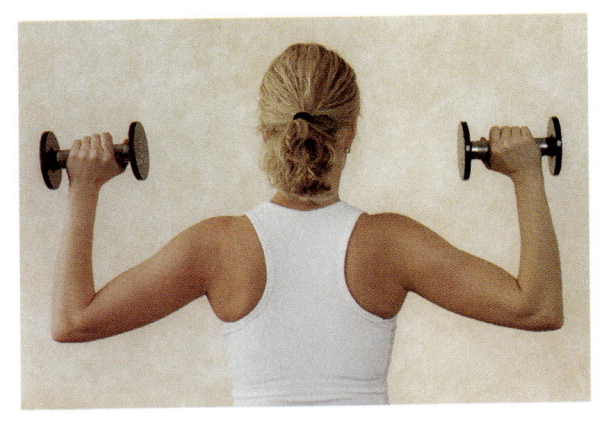

Dumbbell press. Start with a five- to eight-pound weight in each hand. With arms at your sides, bend your arms and raise your hands to shoulder height. Straighten your arms and raise the weights above your head, but still out to the sides. Slowly lower to the starting position. Begin doing three sets of eight to ten reps; work toward three sets of fifteen.

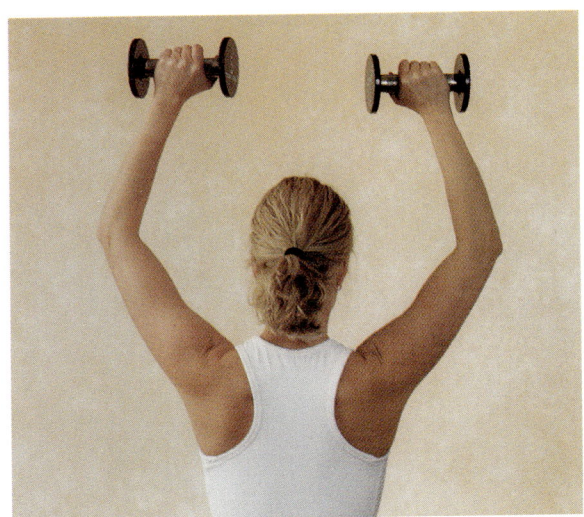

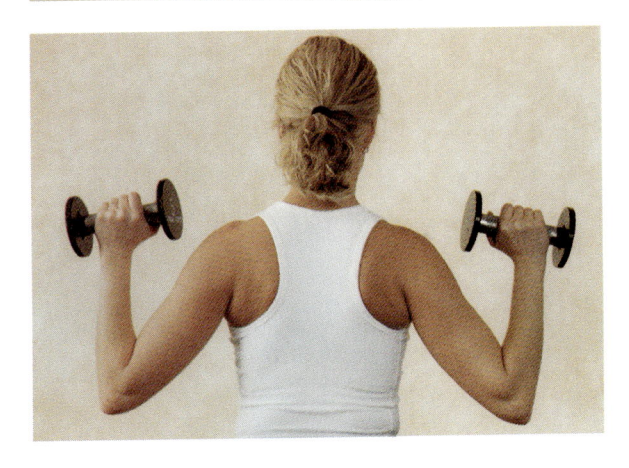

Strength Training

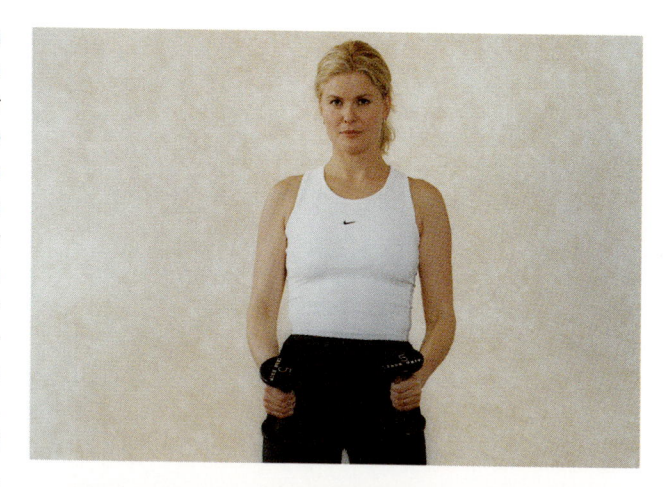

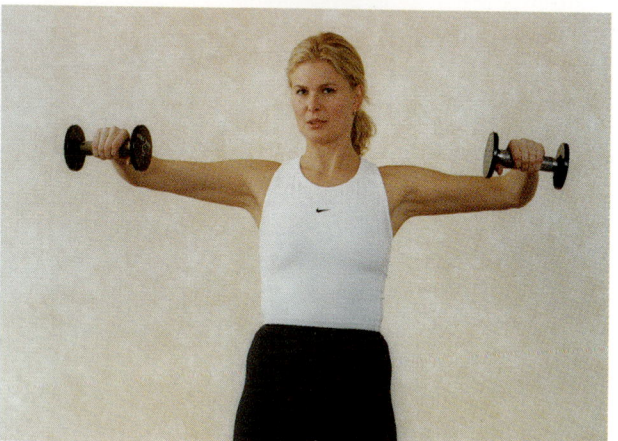

Lateral raise. Start with a weight in each hand, arms down by your sides. Rotate your elbows up so that they're parallel to the floor. Return to the starting position. The key to this exercise is to keep your wrists, elbows, and shoulders in a straight line—don't raise your elbows higher than your shoulders or you'll put too much stress on your wrists and elbows. Again, work toward three sets of fifteen reps.

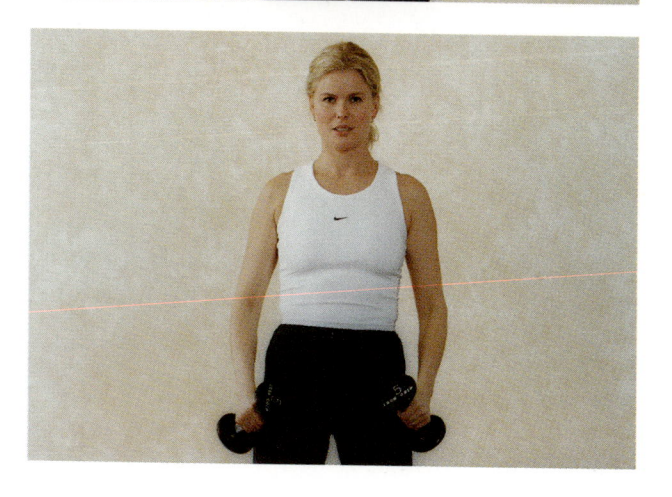

Lateral Raise

Using the same weights, you're going to work your deltoids, or shoulder muscles—key to looking good in a strapless dress!

Upright Row

This is a posture exercise that is really important for women. A lot of new mothers carry their babies on their hip and throw their alignments out. This exercise helps straighten you out, while also working out your upper back and shoulders.

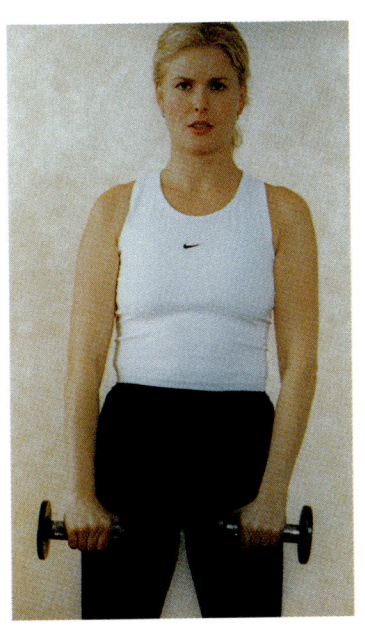

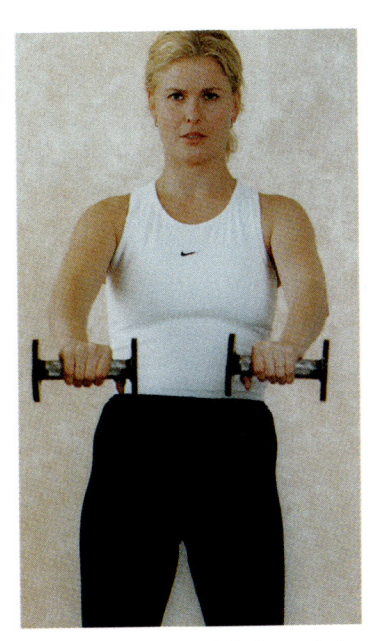

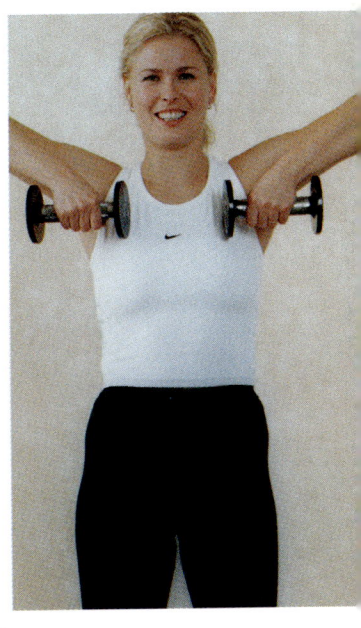

Upright row. Start with your hands by your sides, a weight in each hand. Raise your arms by bending your elbows so that the dumbbells travel up the center of your body, working your elbows up toward your ears (your hands may end up at the sides of your chest, which is fine). Watch out that you don't pull your shoulders up—concentrate on keeping them in a relaxed posture. Work up to three sets of fifteen reps.

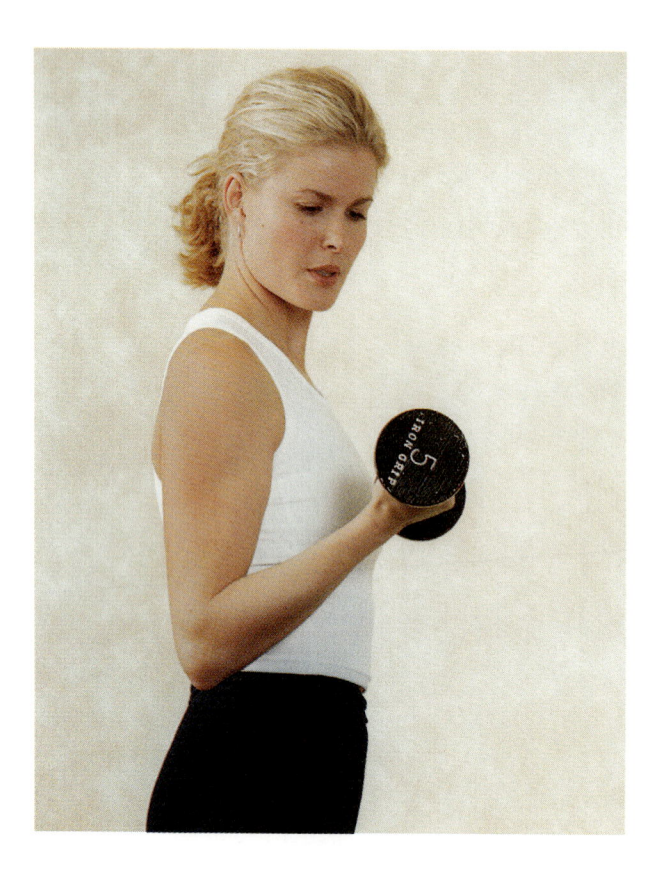

Biceps curls. Begin with a five- to eight-pound weight in each hand, palms facing your thighs. Bend your right elbow, raising your wrist up to your shoulder while rotating your hand so your palm is facing your shoulder. Start with eight to ten reps and work your way up to ten to fifteen, alternating each arm.

Biceps Curls

This is another basic exercise, but the key is to keep your upper arm glued to your side throughout. Move slowly. You don't want to swing or toss the weight. Concentrate on feeling the slow squeezing of your biceps.

One-Armed Dumbbell Press

This is good for your triceps, but it can be a little bit awkward. You must be sure to keep your posture perfectly erect or it can cause some problems.

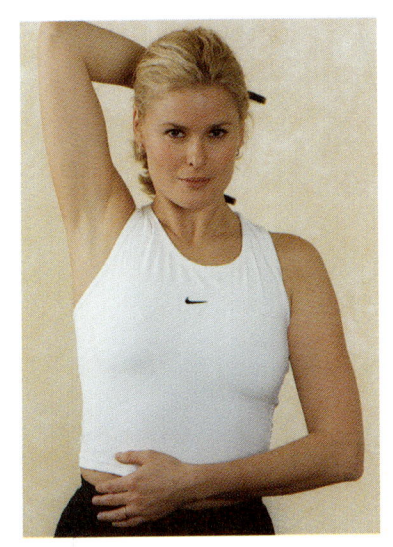

One-armed dumbbell press. Begin with your elbow toward the ceiling and the dumbbell at your ear.

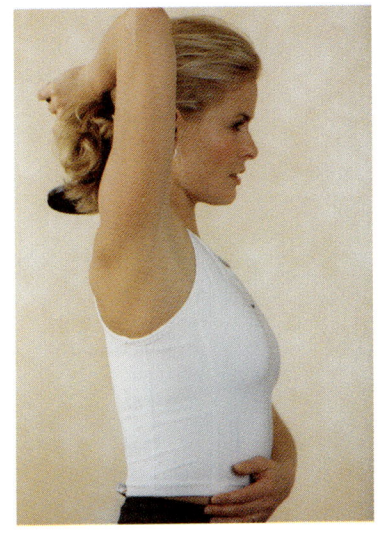

Keep your free hand on your stomach to make sure you're not arching your back.

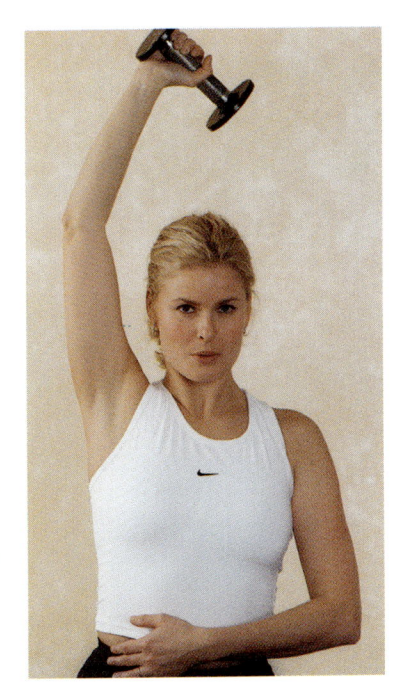

Then extend the weight straight up over your head and slowly return to starting position. Start with eight reps and work up to ten to fifteen.

Strength Training

Diamond Pushups

A safer way to work the same muscles as the one-armed dumbbell press is to do what's called a diamond pushup. Take the same posture as the pushups you did earlier (see page 76), but make a diamond with your thumbs and forefingers, elbows pointed out. There's no chance you can do as many of these as the dumbbell presses, so just do as many as you can. And don't be surprised if your muscles shake—it just means they're tired.

Crunches

On to abdominal work—the part you're probably most interested in. Crunches are one of those exercises that look so easy, but doing them correctly can be hard! One easy way to make sure you don't cheat is to place your legs on a chair so the hip flexor doesn't get involved.

Reverse Crunches

There's almost no motion in this exercise, but it is really effective.

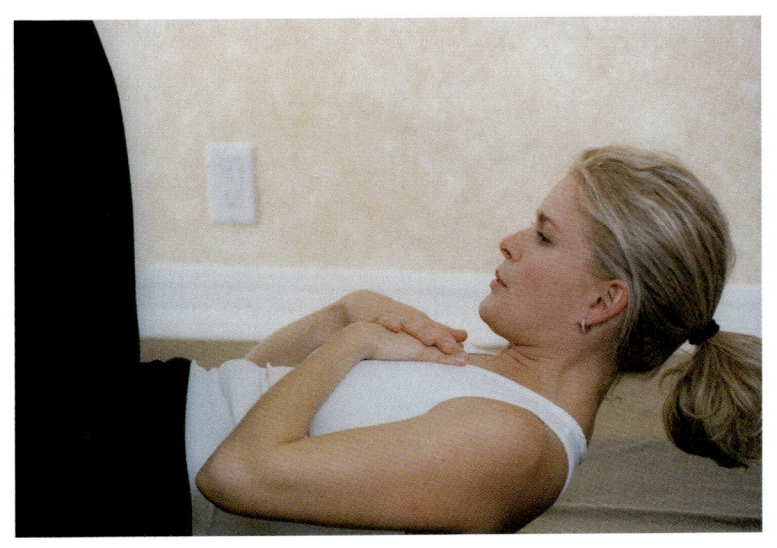

Crunches. Cross your hands across your chest so you don't pull with your arms, and then contract your abdominal muscles. Initiate the movement with your ab muscles, not your upper body—that's just along for the ride. Keep your abs tight and contracted. Your shoulder blades, but not much more of your upper body, should come off the mat. Pause there and then come back down. Don't go too fast, and remember, the goal isn't to sit up, it's to contract those muscles. Do three sets of fifteen to twenty-five reps.

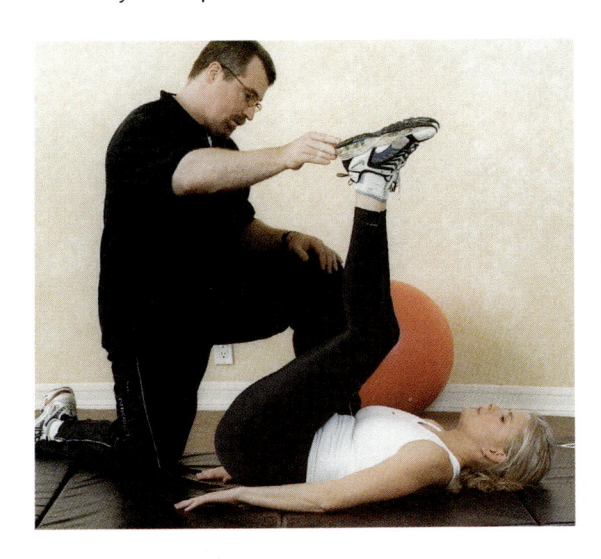

Reverse crunches. Lie on your back with your feet pointing to the ceiling. With your knees pressed together, move them toward your chest, but only three to four inches.

Strength Training

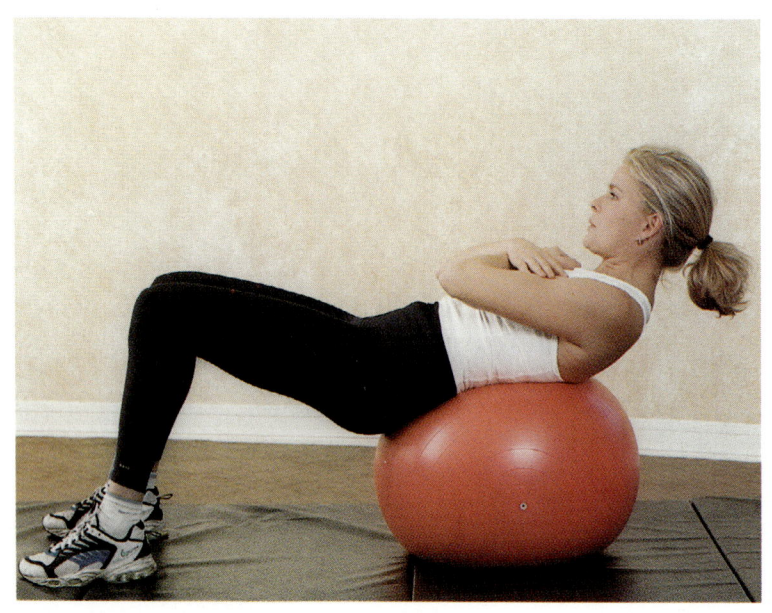

Ball crunches. With the ball in the middle of your back, do the crunch as you would on the floor.

Ball Crunches

This type of crunch is more advanced and gives you more range of motion.

Lower-Ab Ball Crunches

This advanced lower-ab exercise involves strength and balance. Do not try this unless your lower abs are relatively strong.

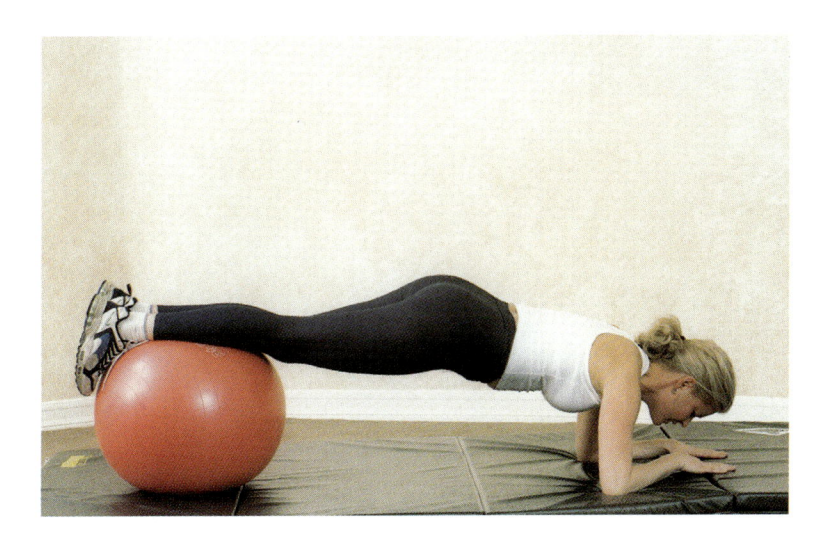

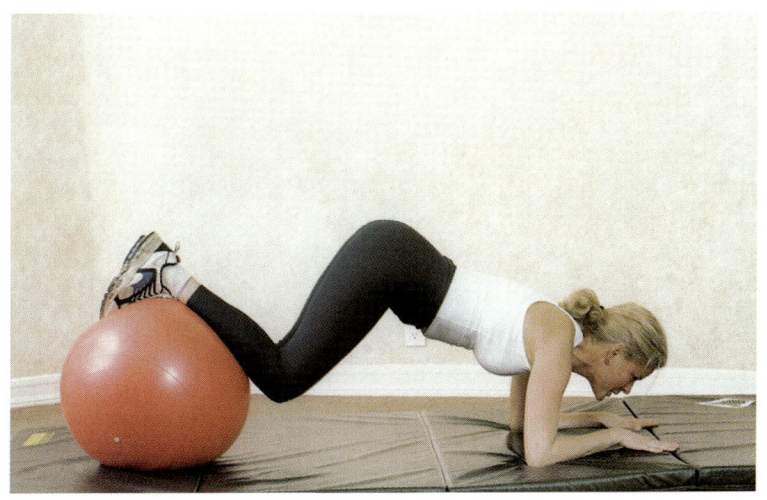

Lower-ab ball crunches. Start in a position similar to a pushup with your elbows on the ground and legs straight but with your feet hooked onto the ball. Then bring your knees slowly into your chest, moving the ball along with them, and then back out. You're probably not going to want to do more than eight to ten, even when you're in great shape.

Strength Training

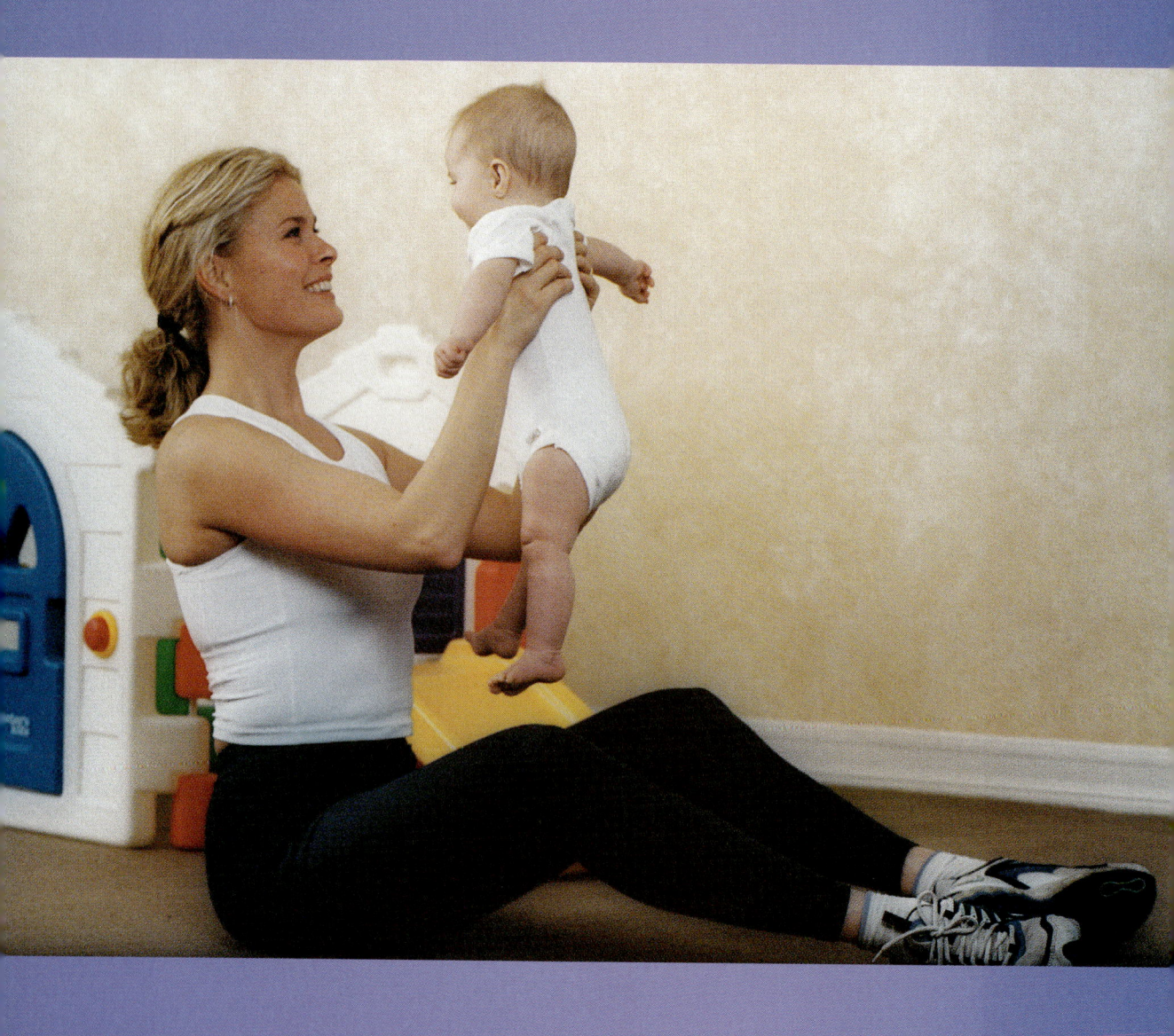

11

Exercising with Your Baby

I know the idea might sound a little silly, but there really are ways to incorporate your baby into your workout routine—and not just by pushing him or her in a stroller while you walk or run, although that's great, too, in the nice weather.

I realized when I had my children that part of our playtime naturally involved me working certain muscle groups. For instance, when you lift your baby above your head, don't you feel it in your arms and back?

Obviously, you want to be careful—you certainly don't want your baby to be uncomfortable! But one night while I was watching my husband do crunches while Hannah sat on his legs and giggled, I saw that there are certain muscle groups that can be worked with your baby. (Believe me, your baby will have more fun than you will!) It's time to spend together, and it can be a good way to physically bond with your child, as well.

EXERCISE FOR LIFE

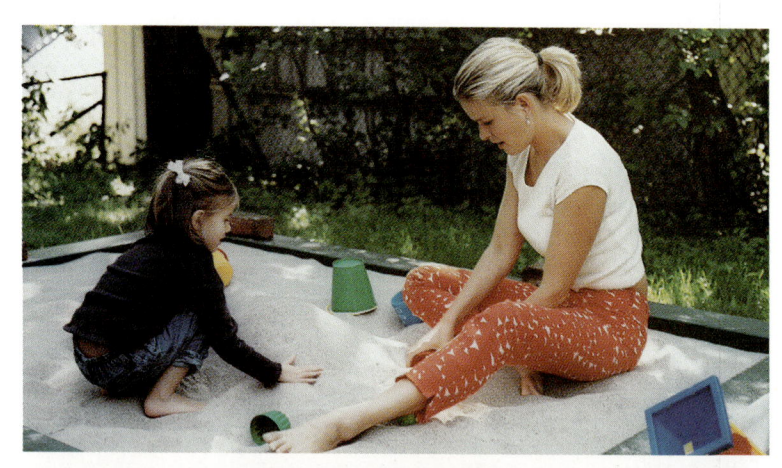

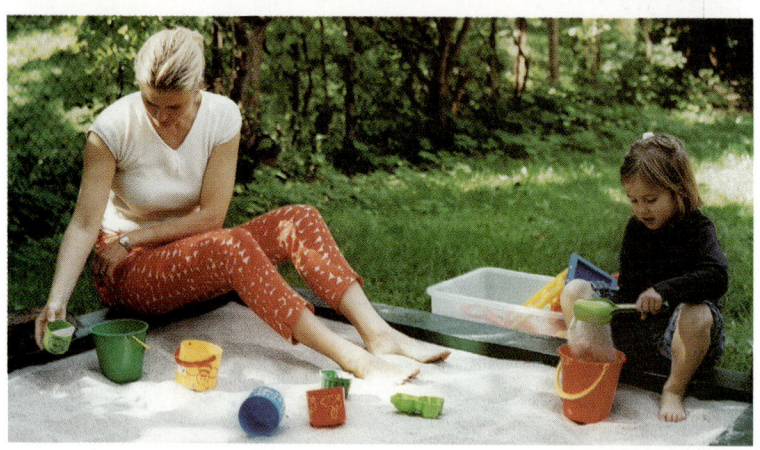

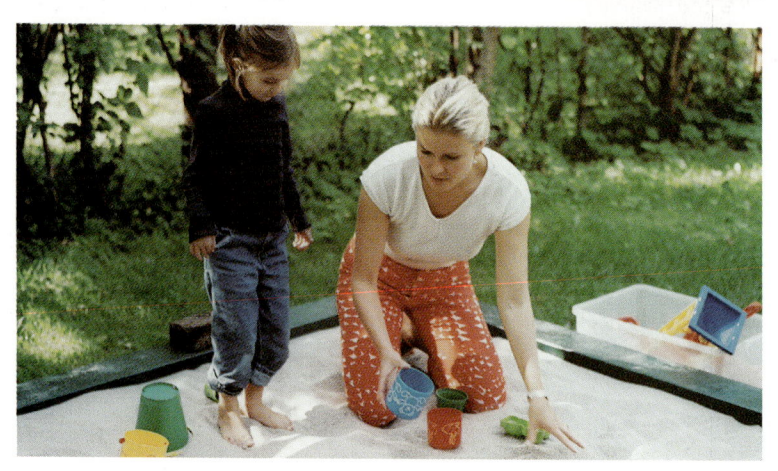

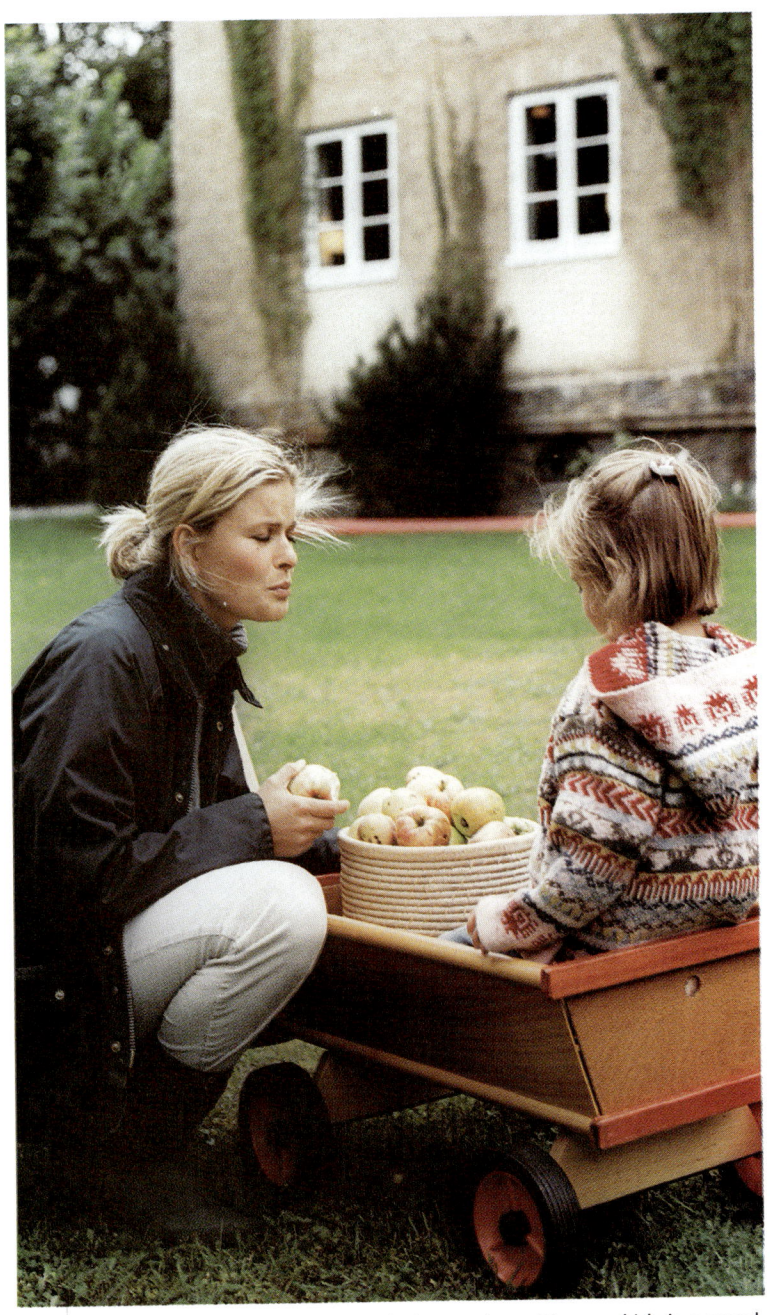

In addition to specific exercises, just being active with your kids is a good way to stay in shape, be a good role model, and have fun together.

Exercising with Your Baby

My trainer, Sean, is against exercising with your baby because you're not concentrating as well as you would be alone, and he points out that a child isn't exactly the proper implement. But if push comes to shove, you can combine a hug with a crunch or a lunge or a squat. Or, lie on your stomach, both you and your baby, and you can raise yourself up into the stretch we covered earlier.

And stretching toward your baby can be a great motivator to get a little farther in the stretch!

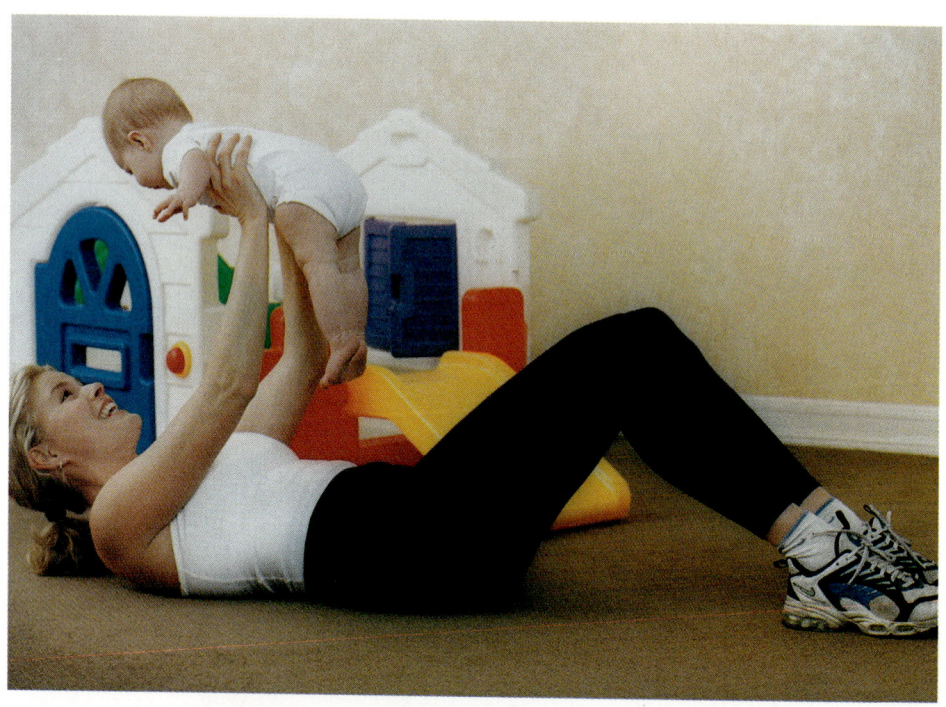

Babies love to "fly" above you. You can turn that into a crunch. Or have baby watch you as you crunch away.

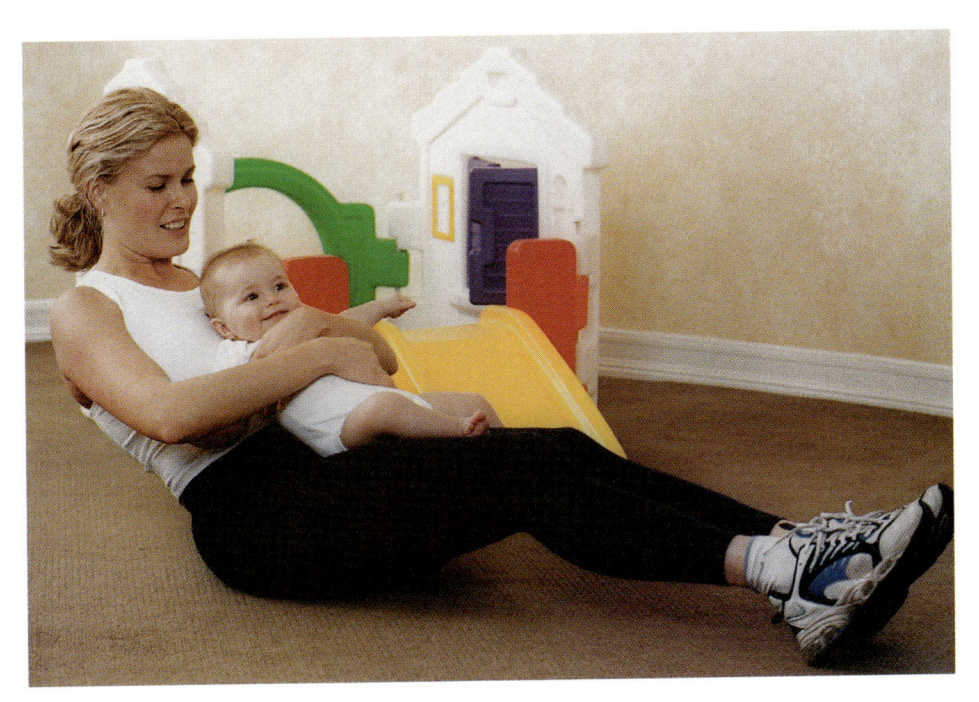

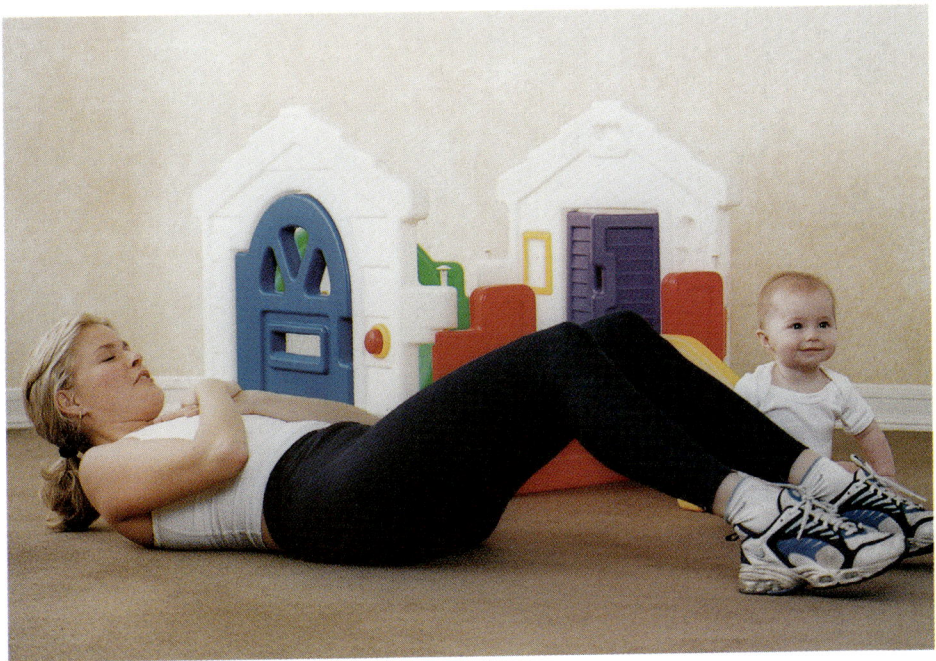

Exercising with Your Baby

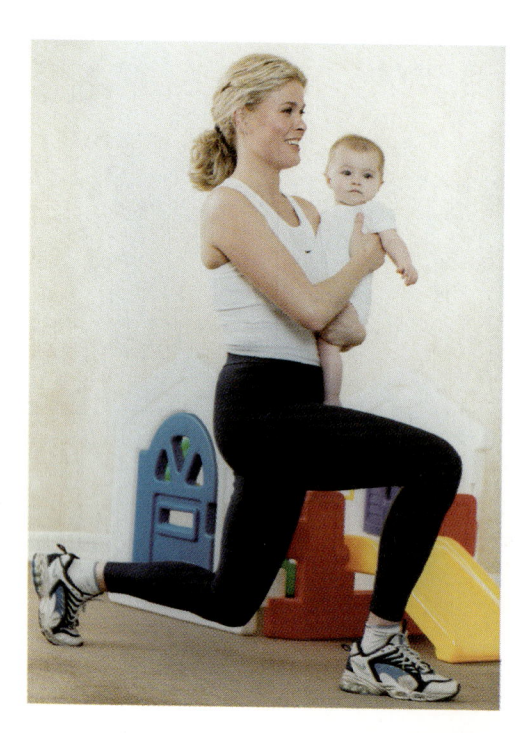

Baby lunges! Be sure to keep your posture correct—back straight and knees no farther out than your ankles.

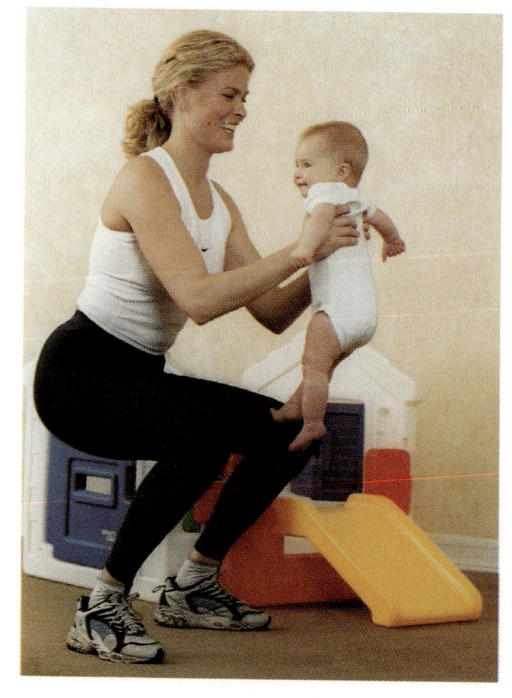

Squats with baby. Again, have fun but be careful to keep proper alignment.

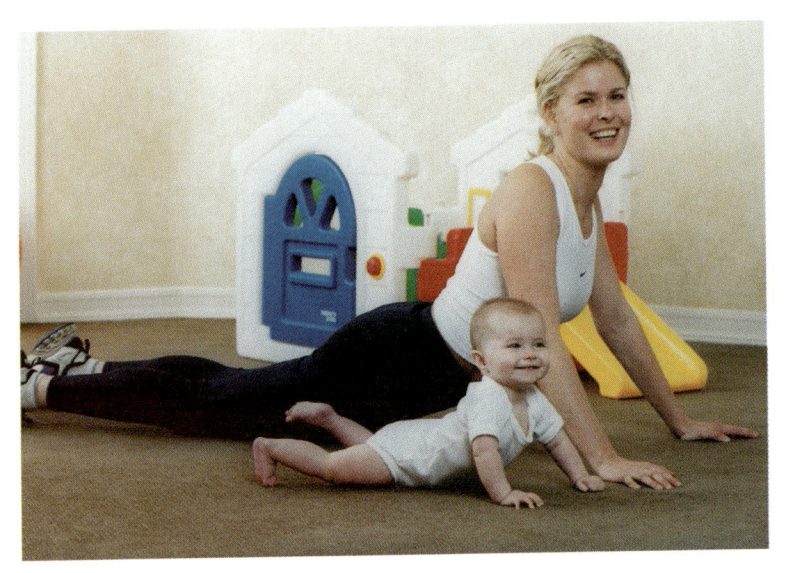

Stretch those abs!

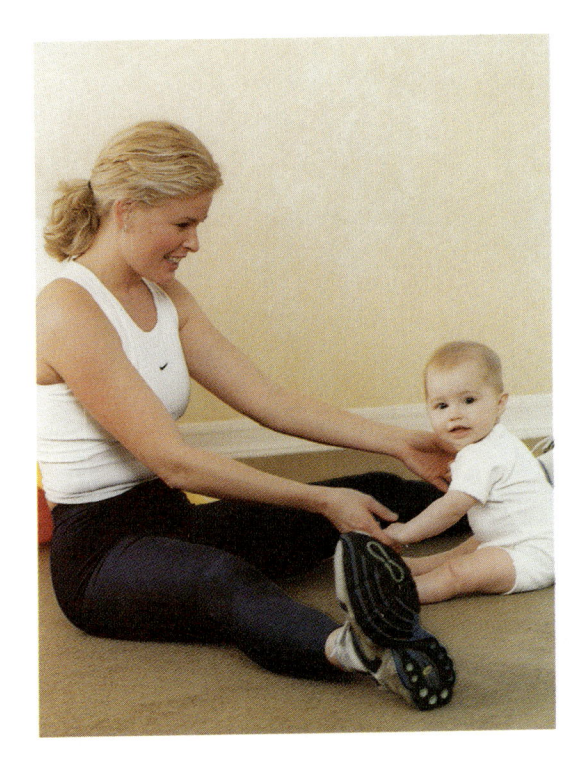

Reach for baby and feel the stretch.

Exercising with Your Baby

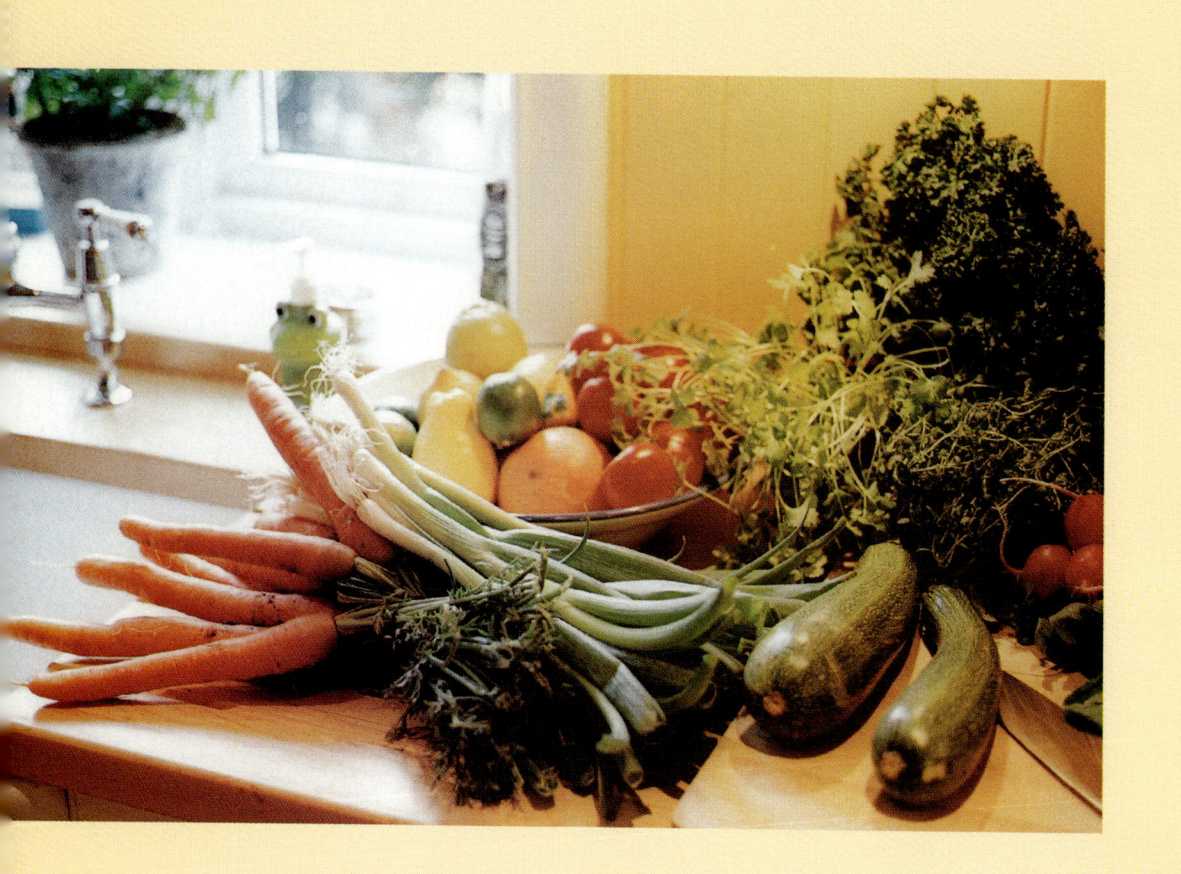

PART THREE

Eating for One Again
Getting the Weight Off

How to eat well, enjoy your food, and not feel deprived and still get back to your fighting weight

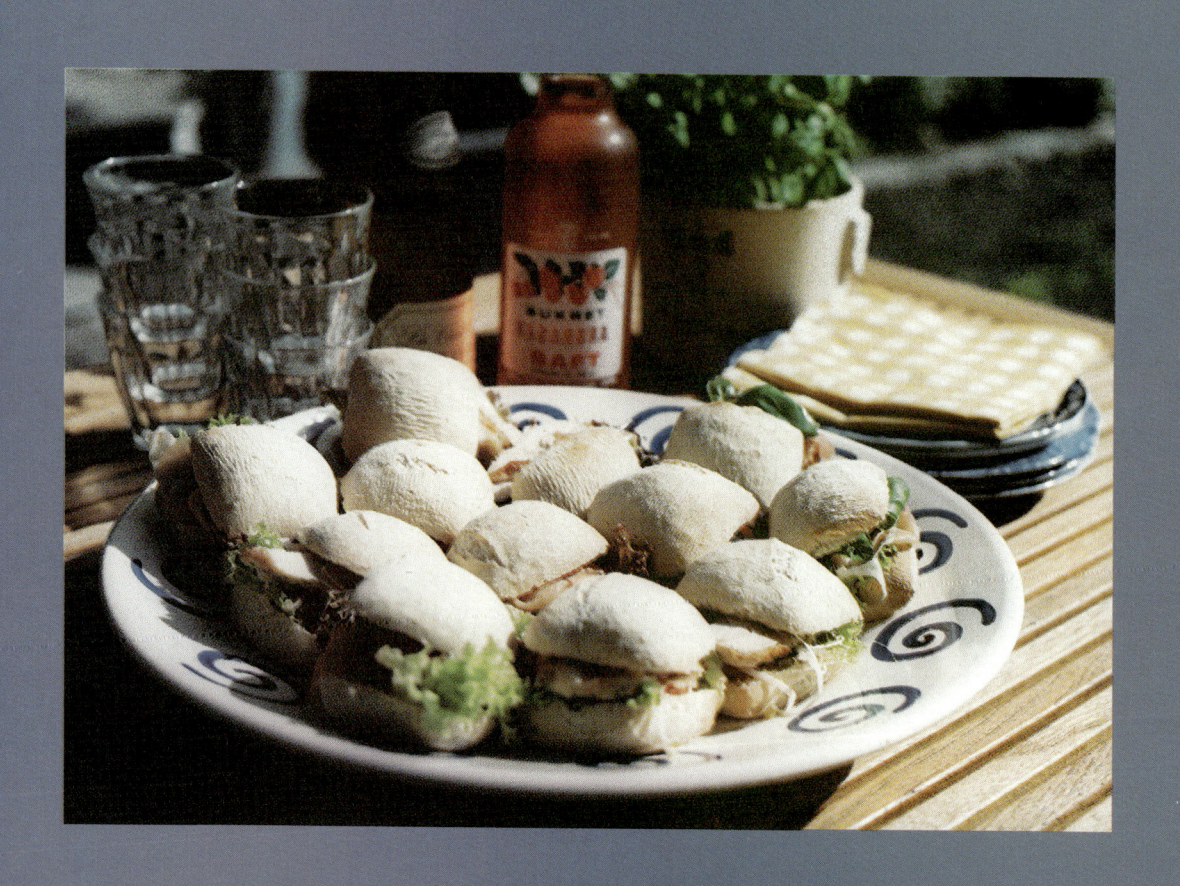

12

Enjoying Your Food

First of all, let me say this again: I do not believe in diets. I eat like a horse. And no, I am not someone who can eat anything I want and not gain weight. But one of the things I've learned is that eating well, and eating healthily, means that *you can be never hungry and still lose weight.*

There's a reason to eat well right now even more important than just to take off a couple of pounds: you need the energy that a healthy eating routine will give you. This is not the time in your life when you need to feel sluggish from carbohydrates. And if you're breast-feeding, you'll also be nourishing your baby, which makes it even more crucial that you eat well.

Now, to me, eating well doesn't just mean having a balanced diet or not overeating. It means enjoying your meals, and it means that what you eat should be wonderful and full of flavor. I'll tell you what you should have in your kitchen and on hand to prepare easy, quick, *delicious* meals, but first, let's talk about how you're going to put more thought into your eating habits—not just for the period it takes to get back to your usual dress size, but for a healthier lifestyle in general.

I always found it amazing when I first came to the States how common it is to see people racing down the street with food in their hands, trying to grab lunch on their way to the next meeting. It was also a culture shock to realize how many people not only eat on the run but also standing up when they're home.

These are behaviors that are totally foreign in Europe, and frankly, one of the reasons I think Europeans tend to be less obese than people in the United States, where an astonishing number of adults are over their healthy body weight. In Europe, it's not that we eat low-calorie, high-protein food all the time, but every meal is concentrated on and enjoyed, even if it's just a sandwich. I think that, mentally, that's really an important aspect to knowing when you're full—how could you possibly feel sated when you spend three minutes stuffing your face at the kitchen counter? We also snack much less frequently in Europe; there aren't vending machines with candy bars in every office building, and people are used to eating nothing between lunch and dinner. That's not because we have smaller appetites. It just means we make the most of the full meals we do have.

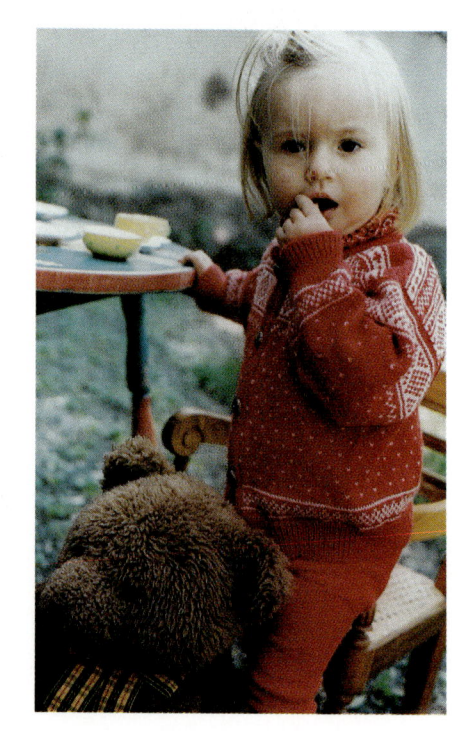

No matter what you're eating—and obviously, I'm not saying you should lounge around for an hour when you grab an apple as an afternoon snack—sit down with the food. Give your body a chance to know it's being fed!

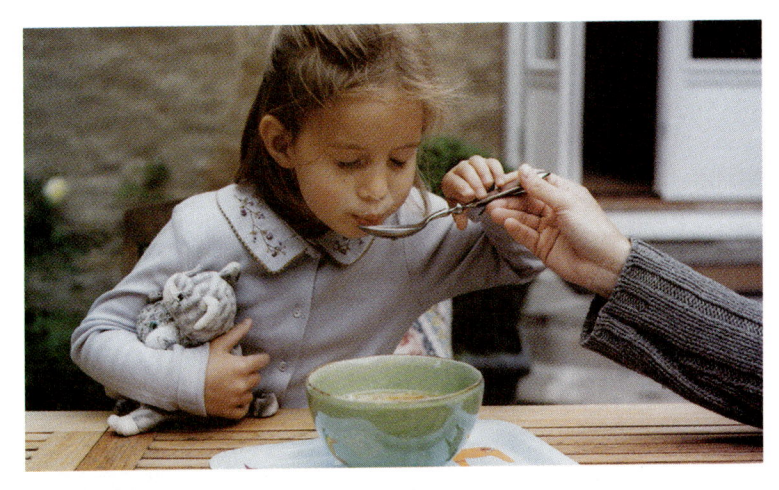

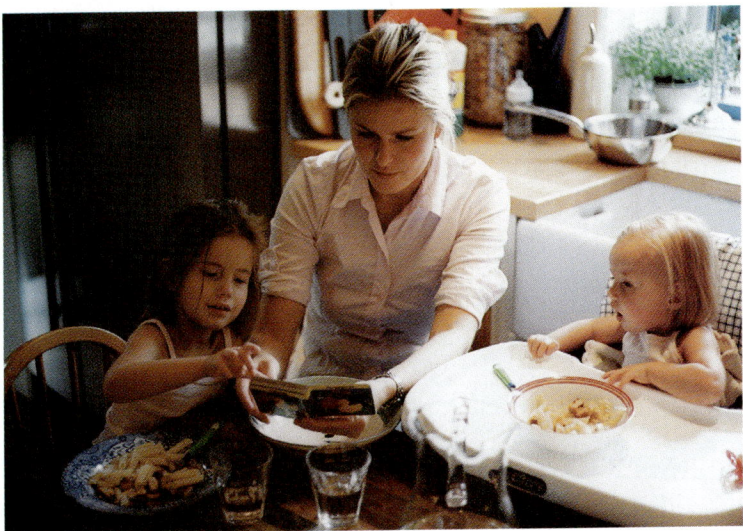

Try to sit down and actually enjoy your food with your kids—or even other adults once in a while!

Enjoying Your Food

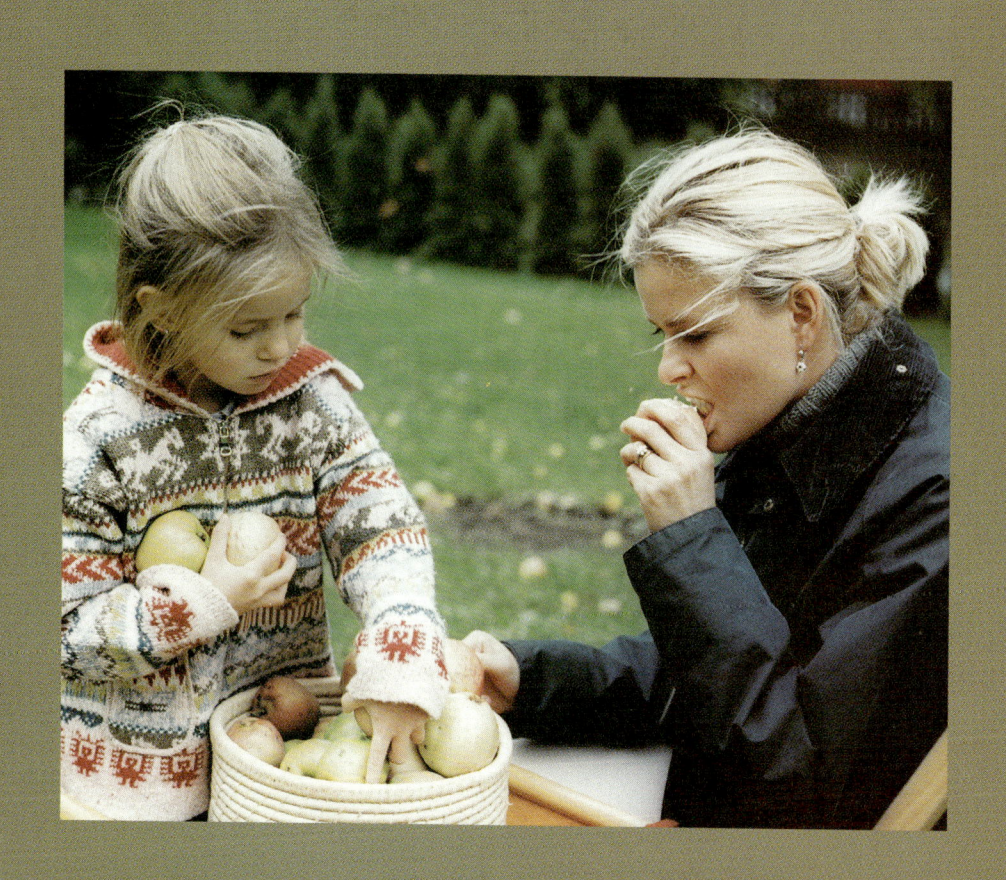

13

Keep Healthy Food— and Only Healthy Food— on Hand!

Especially if you're breast-feeding, you'll have sudden hunger attacks, but being exhausted from your baby's daily needs can make you lunge for the refrigerator too. There's nothing wrong with that—if you're hungry, you should eat. But if you haven't prepared food ahead of time or anticipated that you'll have a need to get something in your stomach in three seconds, that can be where you go wrong. You're likely to grab the closest thing at hand, which is frequently empty calories.

I absolutely allow myself occasional sweets (although I am careful when I'm trying to get the baby weight off not to overindulge). But nobody has ever, ever become overweight because they ate cookies occasionally or had a piece of cake once a week or drank whole milk. Gaining weight—and maintaining a weight gain—comes from overall unhealthy eating.

There's another reason to make sure you're grabbing food that's good for you, and that has nothing to do with the fact that if it's always cookies, your weight will take a bit longer to come off. It's that at this particular time in your life, as you know by now, you need all the energy you can get. Feeding your body is the same as putting fuel in the car; if you fill it with crap right now, you won't have the energy you need to muscle through your day. I can't tell you how much better you'll feel—not just physically, but emotionally as well—if you snack on healthier foods.

In Part Four I'm going to give you some recipes for healthy, easy, and delicious meals, and many of the recipes will include enough for you to have leftovers to snack on. But one trick I find very helpful for the 4:00 P.M. I-need-to-eat-right-this-second attack is to always make sure that I have strips of grilled chicken in the fridge. By cutting them into pieces, I can eat according to my hunger, and I can be sure I'm giving my body the protein it needs.

Again, this is no time to eat less—especially if you're breast-feeding. But you'll be astonished to find how you drop your pregnancy weight just by substituting healthy foods for your usual fast fare, whether its a tuna sandwich on whole wheat in place of chips or a protein bar in place of a Snickers. And because the food is more filling for a longer period of time, you're very likely to find yourself eating fewer wasted calories, without even having to make the effort.

One of the tricks that my trainer, Sean, taught me is to always have nuts and raisins with me. I had always thought of nuts as being very high in fat and calories, but he explained that they're filled with protein and they fill you up fast. You're much less likely to polish off a jar of peanuts than a bag of potato chips. Eating nuts is a perfect example of filling your body with good foods. Something can be low in fat and calories but empty

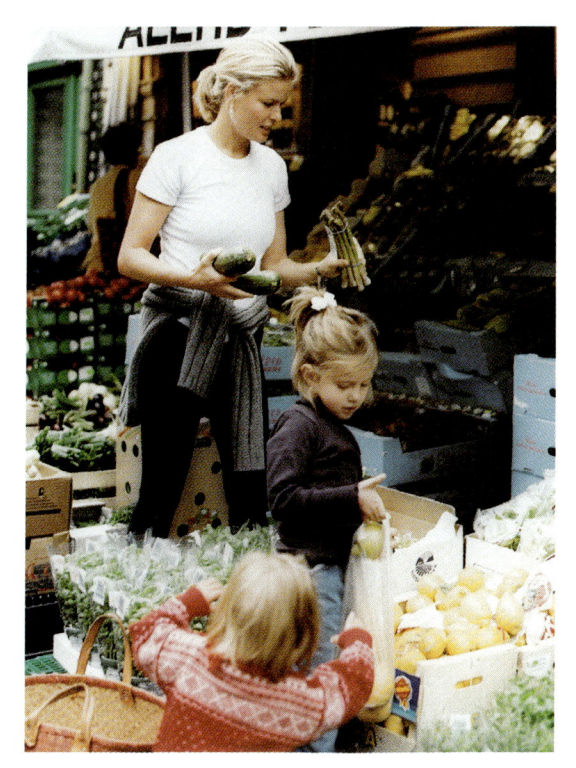

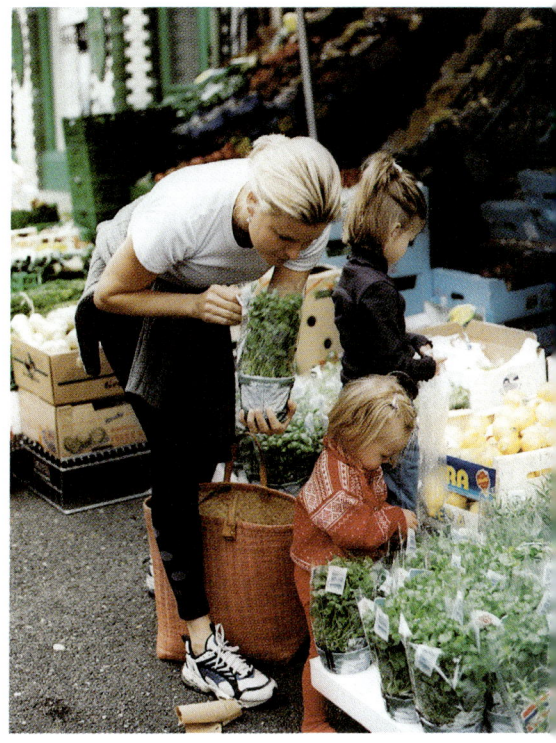

My girls and I make a fun trip out of shopping for fresh, healthy food.

of anything that's good for you, while another food may pack tons of good things into a higher-calorie package.

A point to remember: *if you don't have it, you won't eat it*. This is one of those incredibly simple, obvious, and hard to stick to rules about eating better. Believe me—even though I know it and preach it, there have been numerous times when I've been in the grocery store and thought, "Well, if I buy this bag of cookies, it's really for my daughter," or, "I'll grab this bag of chips and only eat one."

More power to you if you can do it, but I can't! I'm very careful about what I have in the house when I'm carefully watching what I'm eating, because it's too easy to fall into the cookie jar, as it were. Now, I certainly don't want to deprive my children of treats, so I do buy them sweets, but I make sure to buy them *their* favorite cookies, which luckily aren't the ones that appeal to me.

Also, I think it's helpful if your children can see you snacking healthily, because then they'll do it naturally. So often when I'm in the park with my kids, I see that mothers aren't eating, but they're feeding their kids chips and chocolate, as if they're allowing their children to eat everything they won't allow themselves to eat. Julia loves cucumbers, and she'll never think of them as "boring" or something she has to eat. Vegetables and nuts will never be an unacceptable substitute to cookies or candy.

On the same note, insist that your children sit while they're eating as well, and you sit with them. Don't turn on the TV or talk on the phone. Even if it's five minutes, you're instilling in your kids the importance, both socially and health-wise, of making a meal out of food.

In terms of your own eating, just remember, when you're absolutely starving, you're not going to run out to the store for a pint of ice-cream—that might actually take time! You're going to grab what you see in your refrigerator or on your shelves. If you're going to pay attention to the food, look for the amount of protein in it before you glance at the fat content.

When we get to the section on cooking (see Chapter 16), I'll tell you what you should have in your kitchen in terms of preparing meals, but let's first discuss snacks. There are certain things you should make sure you're always stocked up on. Again, don't think of it in terms of what you can't eat—that's self-defeating, and, as I said earlier, there's nothing you can't eat in moderation. Instead, pay attention to the things that you should eat, the things that are good for you and will help keep you going—such as bags of nuts and raisins.

I'm not a big fan of peanut butter, probably because I didn't grow up with it, but if you like it, a tablespoon of it can be a wonderful, stick-to-your-ribs snack. Put it on a piece of apple or a rice cake and you have an instant treat. (If you can stay away from a lot of pastas and breads during this period, that's very helpful; they will make you feel sluggish and hungry sooner than something high in protein like peanut butter.)

I also make sure to always have fruit and vegetables on hand. I'm not going to tell you to "treat" yourself to an apple as a snack, because if I read that, I would immediately feel like I was on some cruel "Survivor"-like "diet." But it's helpful to be able to grab an apple and throw it in your purse while you're running out the door, just in case you find yourself out somewhere and starving. It will hold you over until you get something else in your stomach, and you'll grab for that, especially if it's already in your bag, before you go buy a candy bar.

In addition, make sure to fill your refrigerator with things like yogurt—it's very filling and very good for you. If you put honey and fruit in plain yogurt, you'll have a sweet-tasting, almost dessert-worthy treat on hand! And as I said, I always make sure to have pieces of chicken and fish. The best trick for accomplishing this is to take out an extra chicken breast when you're preparing a meal for your family and stick it under the broiler. Then, cut it into strips and put it away for later!

Don't feel defeated if you find yourself eating more than ever. Especially when I'm breast-feeding, I'm hungrier than I've ever been, and I find myself eating even more than my husband. (I also need to eat in the middle of the night when I'm up with the kids, but I try to watch the chocolate.) But as I've said, it's not the amount that counts, it's what the amounts are of.

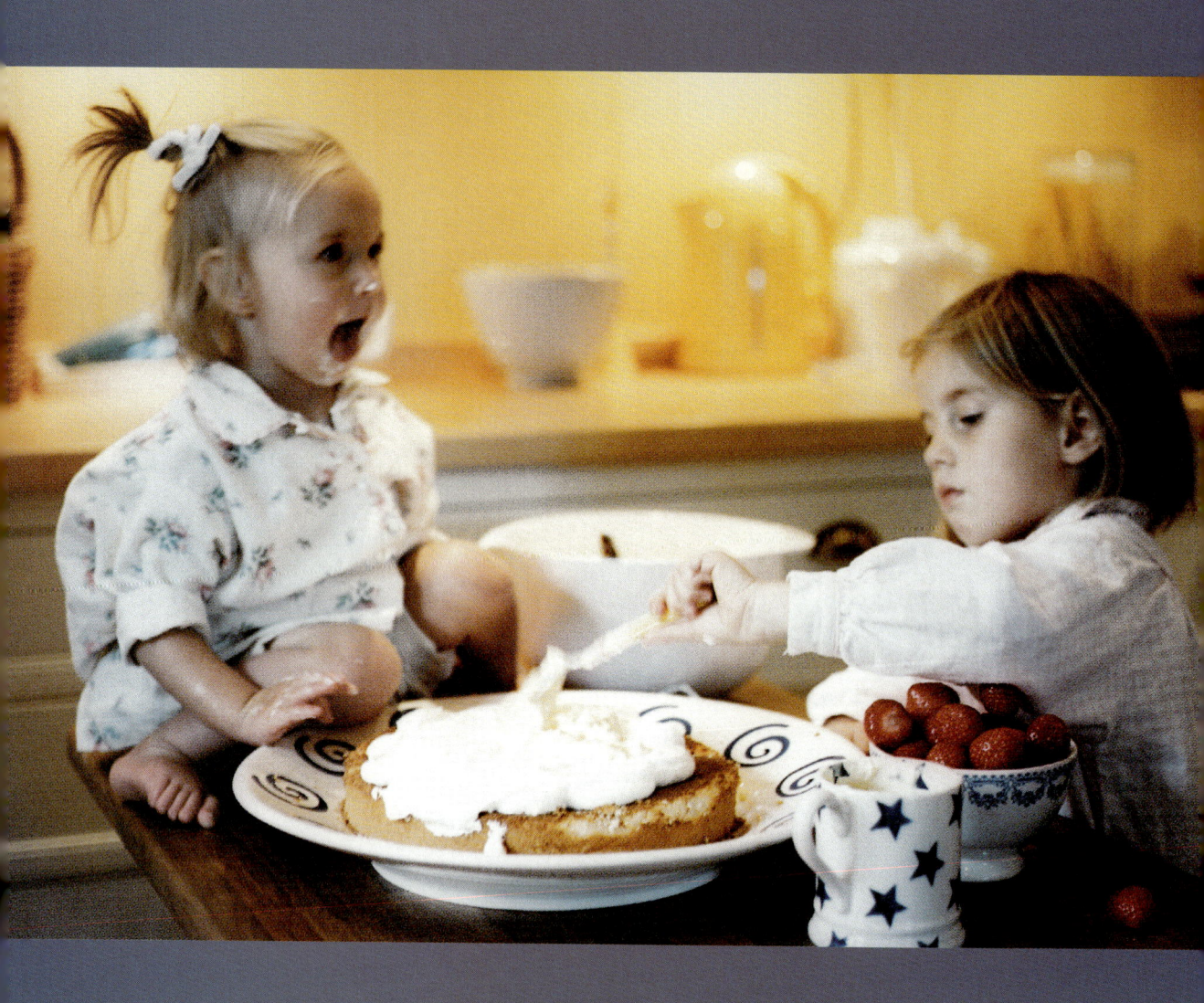

14

Indulge Yourself!

OK, so now you've got your kitchen filled with great food, we've got you sitting down for your meals, and you're snacking on fuel-filled things that will get you to your next meal. But what about a treat every now and then?

Go for it! There's not a weight-watching plan in the universe that will work if you walk around feeling miserable and punished. Maybe you'll be able to do it for six weeks, but then you'll fall off the wagon. There is nothing wrong with treating yourself now and then. It's just like when I told you that I give myself five free passes a week when I don't have to go to the gym, even though I've scheduled it. Not going then doesn't mean I've stopped exercising; it means that I've incorporated exercise into its rightful place in my life.

It's the same thing with food. Food is meant to give you pleasure, and this is no time to deprive yourself of a quick hit of pleasure occasionally! My husband is addicted to chocolate and found that he was putting on weight, so now he tells himself that he can eat chocolate on Saturdays. That way he eats less of it, but he's not feeling deprived during the week because he knows his date with the cocoa is coming soon.

I tend to be less regimented about what I eat, although I think that it's a great idea to take one day a week to eat as you please. Trust me—you're not going to start with an entire pizza for breakfast and then go through all the food groups until midnight. But it can work very well if you tell yourself that you don't have to worry about it one day a week.

For me, what works best is choosing how I'm going to treat myself. If I'm out for a cup of coffee and I see a piece of carrot cake I have to have, I don't sit there and obsess about it. I allow myself to get it, and then I'll eat part of it. Because I feel like I've treated myself by getting it and having some, I don't feel like I'm punishing myself by not finishing it. The point is, don't make it an issue. That's when you'll binge like a rebellious child who has been told she can't have something, instead of an adult who can judge what's best for herself.

It's amazing how your brain works—once you tell yourself you can have something, you tend to approach the situation (or in this case, a piece of carrot cake!) with a lot more respect for yourself. If I worried that I couldn't have it, I would eat the entire piece. But because I know I can, and it will be there, I'm more comfortable eating half of it. That said, I do then try to cut back a bit on the other end of the day, because otherwise I feel disappointed with myself, which means, as you know, eating even more! Another easy way to think about it when you're out for dinner is you can have a glass of wine, or you can have a piece of bread. Again, you're making a choice—you are not a victim—and you can have what you want. It's just that right now, you can't have *everything* you want. Here's the thing to remember: *you are not depriving yourself—you are making choices.*

The trick here is very, very simple. The way you're eating now, just like they way you're exercising, is about empowering *you*. It's about feeling better, more in control, and healthier. Setting yourself up to binge is self-defeating to all of this. Imagine how proud you'll be if you can treat yourself and then stop after a few bites! That said, if you feel like you're too tired to stop after a few bites, here's my last resort trick: *throw it out.*

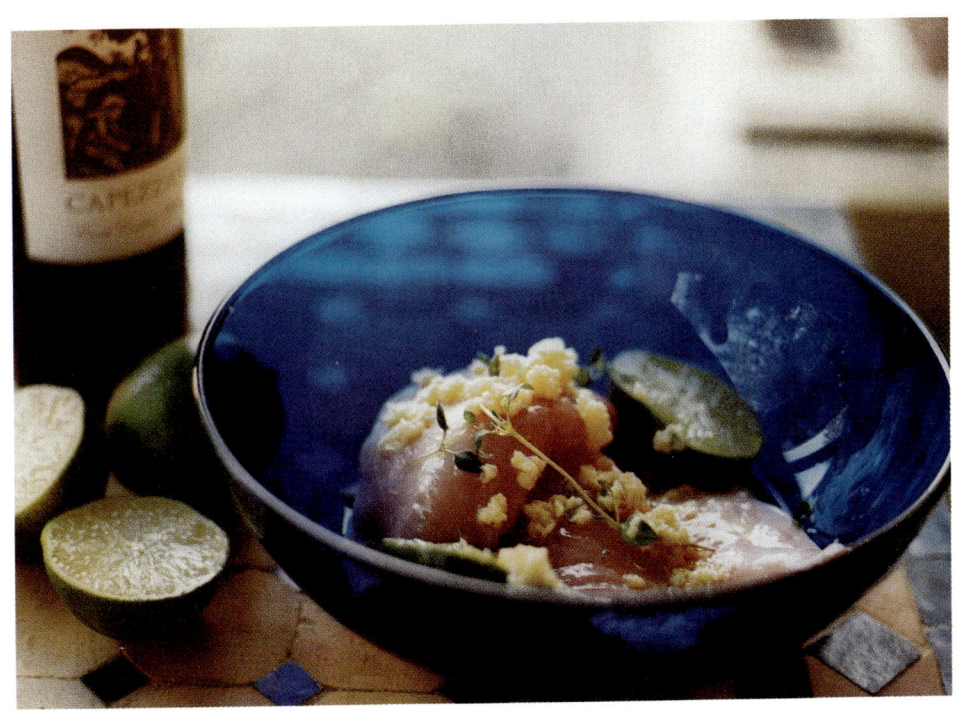

There's nothing wrong with an occasional glass of wine with your meal—just go easy on the bread in exchange.

Indulge Yourself!

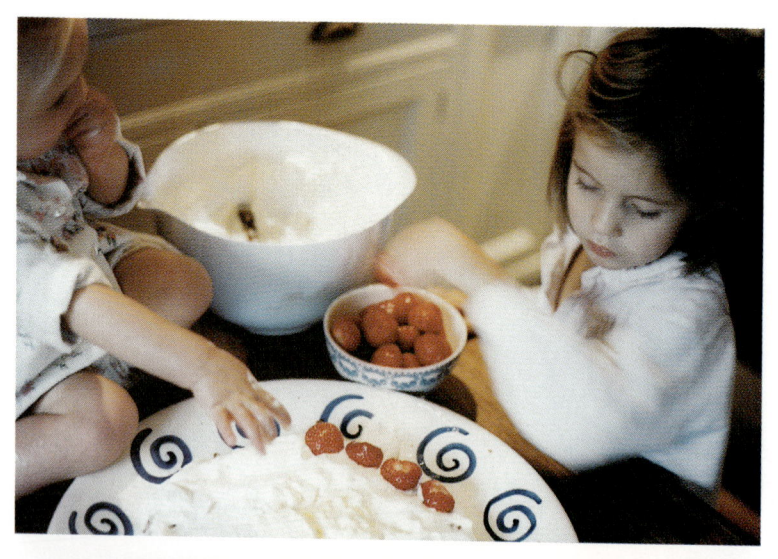

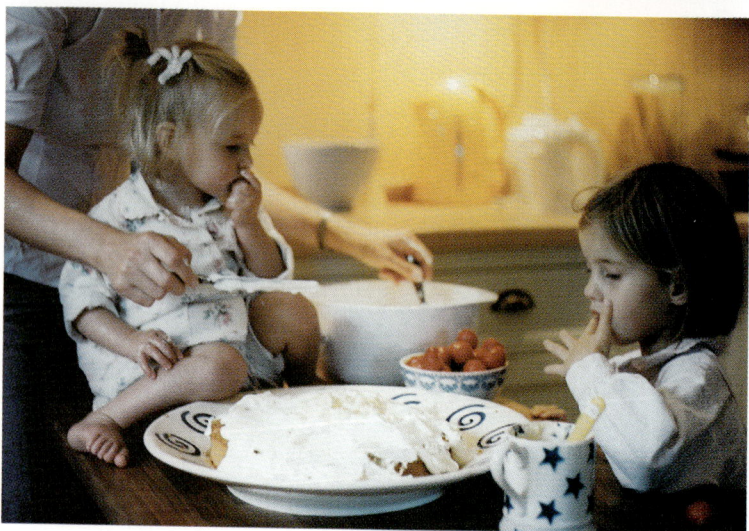

When you can, select indulgences that are somewhat healthy—like perfectly ripened fruit. Let the kids have the cream!

I don't usually crave sweets, but after I had Hannah and Julia, I was a crazy woman for chocolate. There was a period in there where I really couldn't trust myself, so I would get in the habit of buying a chocolate bar, eating half, and then immediately throwing the other half out—and not somewhere where it could easily be fished out!

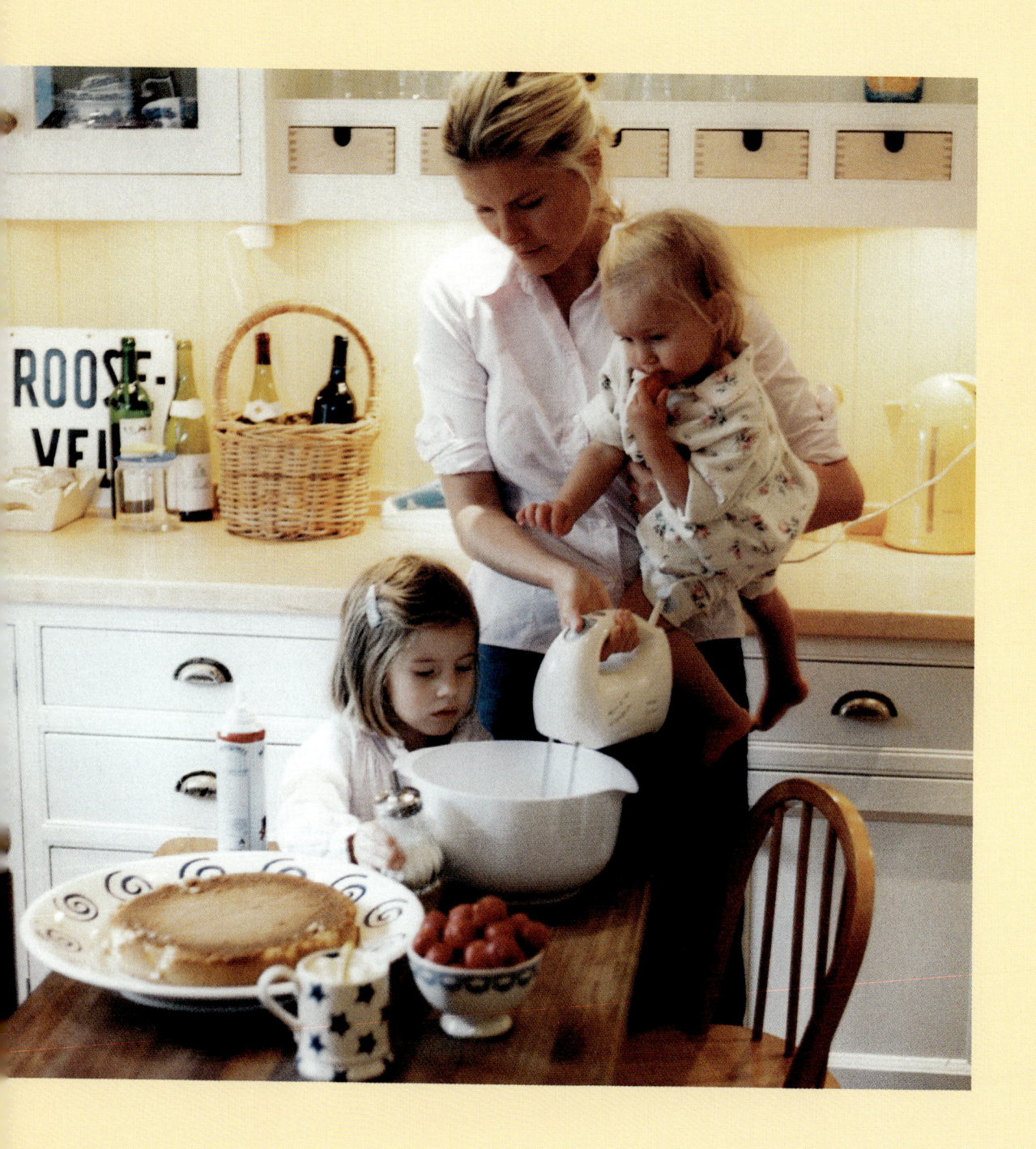

PART FOUR

Cooking for the Whole Family

Suggestions and recipes for my favorite healthy foods along with ways to adapt them for the whole family to enjoy

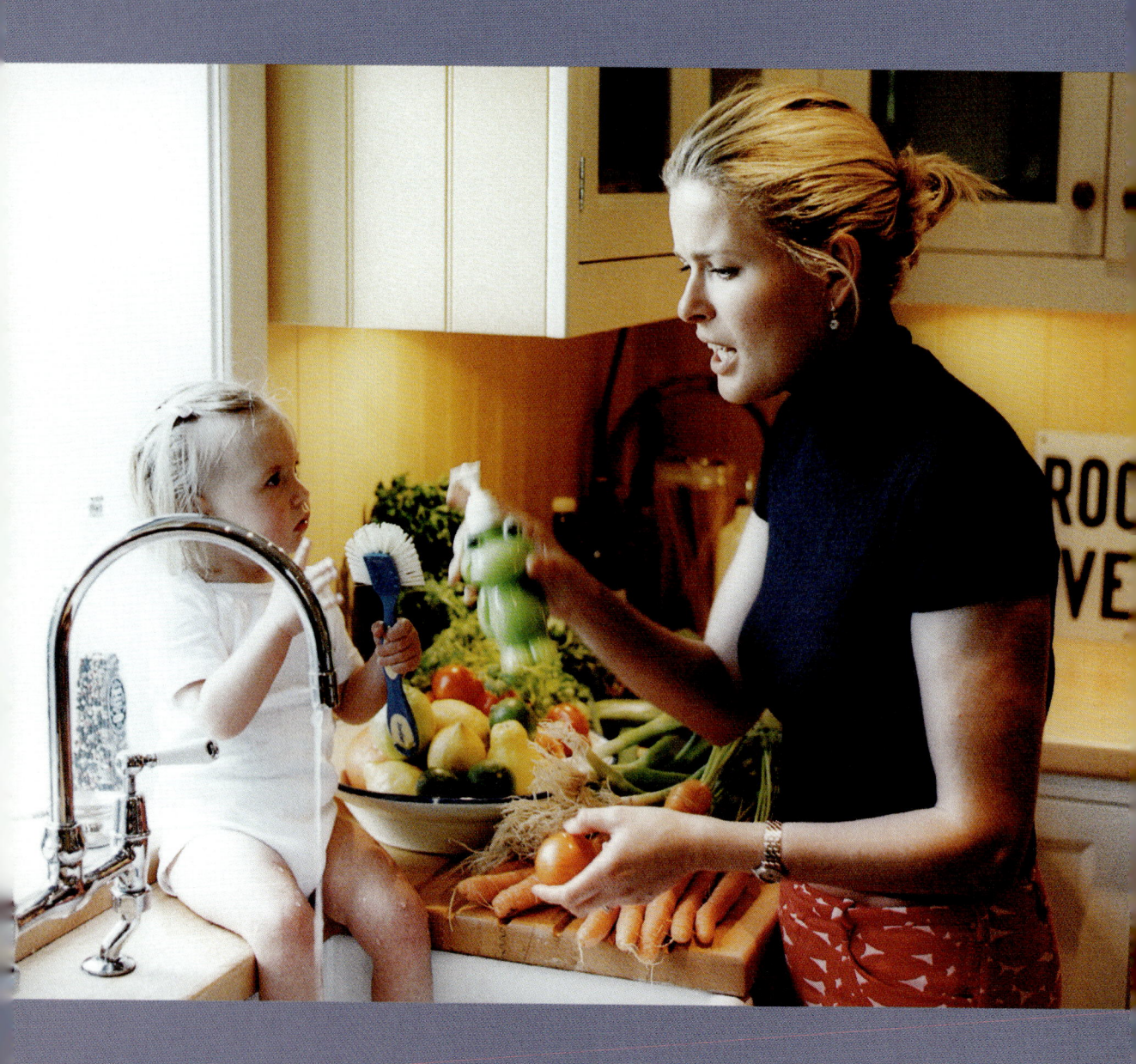

15

Cooking for Two and a Half

I've always loved to cook and have found, when comparing myself to my noncooking friends, that it's much easier to eat healthful meals when you're preparing them yourself. Plus—and this is vital right now—because you can adjust them to exactly the way you like, you're more likely to feel satisfied! But if, like me, you have a toddler as well as an infant (and if you don't yet, that infant will be a toddler before you know it!), you're not in a position to focus on just cooking "healthy" meals for yourself. You have to make food that your child will enjoy and that's good for her too.

The recipes I've included here can all be cooked quickly. The ingredients are easy to get, and as for the herbs and spices, I'm going to give you a list of things to always have in your kitchen. And the best thing is that many of the recipes will provide leftovers, can be frozen, or will be even better two days after you make them.

I am a strong, strong believer that if your food is flavorful, you will eat less and be more satisfied, so to that end, I advocate cooking with olive oil. Again, people aren't overweight because they drizzle their fish with virgin olive oil—they're overweight because they constantly eat foods *fried* in oil. The flavor of good olive oil is irreplaceable, and olive oil has been shown to be "good" fat, rather than bad. Believe me—a salad tossed with a bit of beautiful oil, balsamic vinegar, and salt and pepper will taste delicious; without it, you'll feel like a rabbit!

The recipes I'll give you in the following chapter should provide meals to satisfy everyone, but there are a few shortcuts that will help you balance both your needs and your child's. For instance, consider simple ways in which you can prepare both you child's meal and yours with the same foods, but then slightly alter the way they're cooked. Julia loves eggs in the morning for breakfast, and for her, there's nothing wrong with having them every day. But for me, when I'm trying to eat more protein and fewer calories, it's not necessarily the best way to start the day every day.

But I can cook for us together very simply: I make Julia an omelet or scrambled eggs with cheese, and when it comes to my own, I leave out the cheese and one egg yolk, which has protein but is high in calories (I do always still cook my eggs in a little butter, because I love the flavor). Also, make a list of foods that are good for you and your child, foods that you both enjoy. Julia loves oatmeal, which is a great breakfast for me too when I'm watching my weight. But while Julia likes it with maple syrup and a little cream, I'll put fruit and a sprinkle of brown sugar or a little honey on mine.

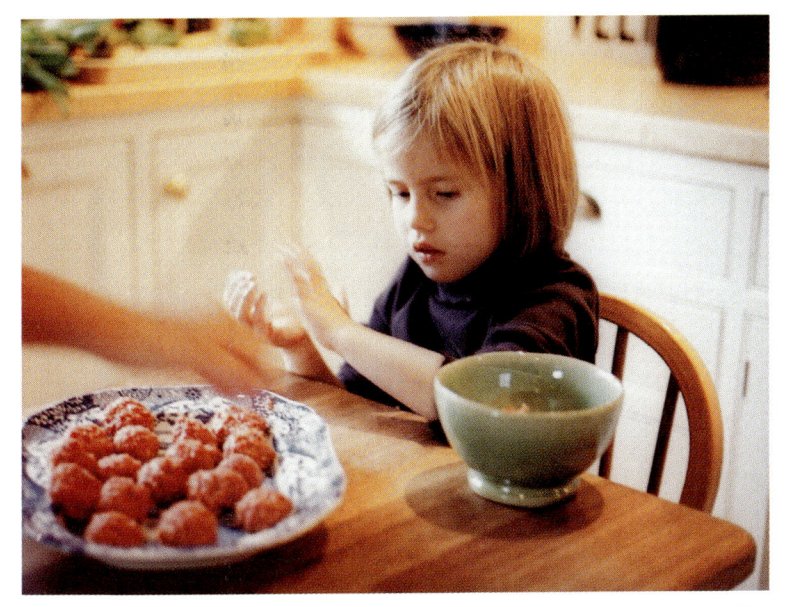

Letting older kids help in the kitchen is a great way to pass on your healthy eating habits. And it's fun for the kids too.

Something I feel very strongly about, especially living in the world of modeling where so many women have eating disorders, is that I don't pass any unhealthy eating habits onto my children. My mother taught me that food is a vital part of enjoying life and is your friend, and my children should learn that from me as well. It's important that Julia and Hannah see me eating, and not just playing with lettuce leaves but really enjoying what I eat. Meals for us are family time. It's a daily celebration and a time to be grateful for what we have, especially each other. It's about sharing our company, not counting calories.

I never want Julia to be aware that I'm eating less than usual. The fact that for a few months I grill my fish with lemon

Cooking for Two and a Half

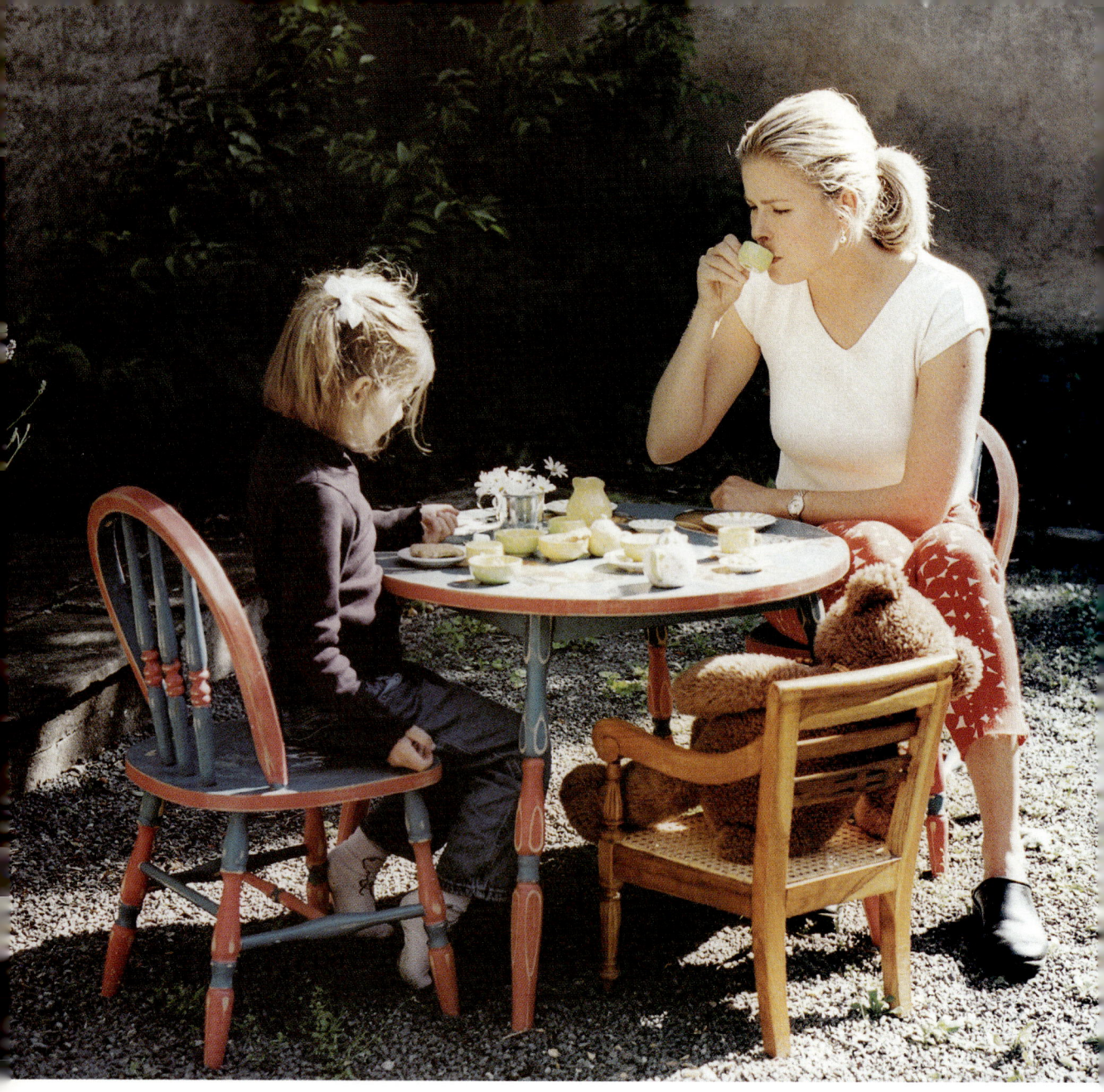

It's important to me that my daughters see me enjoying healthy foods and not obsessing about dieting.

Cooking for the Whole Family

and olive oil while I bread hers is something far too subtle for a child to notice. And Julia loves potato salad made with yogurt as much as with mayonnaise. So we can still enjoy meals as family time, and we can eat the same things, with just a few alterations.

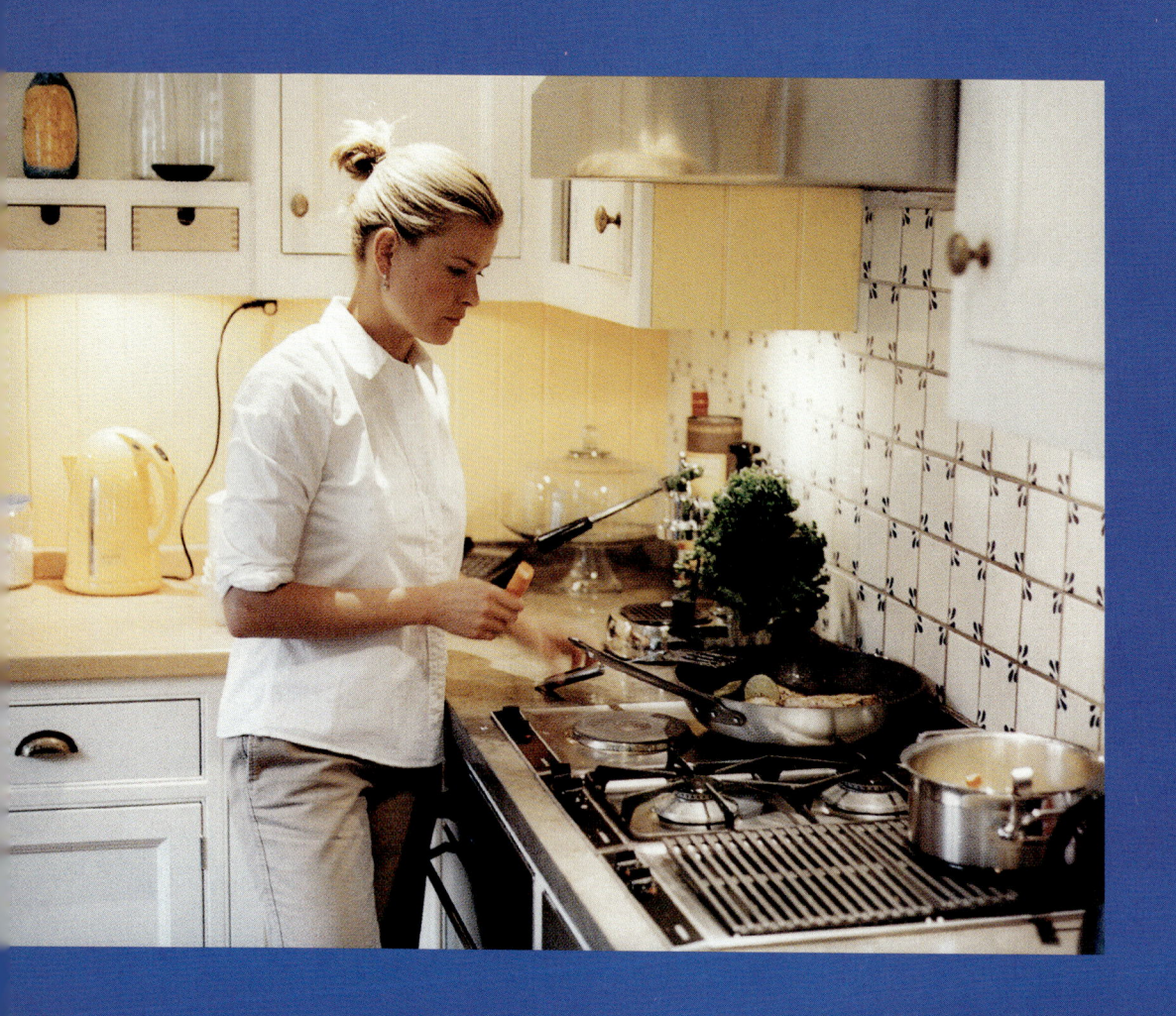

16

My Favorite Healthy Recipes

If you have the items in the list below on hand, you'll be able to transform the simplest foods—with total ease—into delightful dinners using the recipes contained in this chapter.

Take this list to the grocery store and stock up:

- **Virgin olive oil.** Splurge on a virgin olive oil that's flavorful. A little bit of a wonderful oil can go farther than a bland one poured on.

- **Balsamic vinegar.** You'll use it on salads and as a low-calorie, highly flavorful marinade.

- **Soy sauce.** Again, this is a low-calorie, highly flavored item you can use for dressings and marinades.

- **Plain yogurt.** Be sure to get a large container. Not only is it a great snack with some jam or jelly in it, but it's also an easy and healthy way to add flavor when you're cooking.

- **Fresh ginger.** Grab a piece of this tasty herb. By grating it into sauces and marinades, you will add punch to dressings and marinades for meat, chicken, and fish.

- **Fruits and veggies.** Stock up on apples, carrots, and fresh vegetables that you won't mind snacking on raw.

- **Lemon.** Always have lemon in your fridge for adding flavor to your food.

After you've stocked up on these staples, you should upgrade your spice rack. Having a well-stocked spice rack will be the difference between a bland piece of grilled chicken and a fabulous chicken curry. It's also one of the easiest things you can do for your kitchen, because in one trip to the grocery store, you can stock up on a month's worth of flavor. So, hit the spice rack and grab:

- Dried basil
- Cumin
- Curry
- Herbs de Provence
- Yellow mustard seeds
- Paprika
- Dried parsley
- Red pepper flakes
- Dried rosemary

Herbs de Provence is a mixture of herbs sold at most supermarkets in the spice department, but if it's not at yours, mix up a little dried rosemary, oregano, marjoram, and thyme and store it in a container. This is ideal for everything from flavoring eggs and chicken to putting on pasta without adding too much salt.

This selection will do the trick, but if your grocery store sells fresh herbs, I recommend grabbing a few fresh plants. You can keep them on your windowsill and pick them as you need. I make sure to always have basil and rosemary plants to make easy pestos, roasted chickens, and more.

Now your kitchen is set to make easy, healthy meals you'd pay a lot to have in restaurants! The next section has some of my favorite dishes to cook for family and friends using the ingredients above. And if they just happen to be good for me and low in fat and calories, nobody but I would know!

The Recipes

These recipes are to get you back in the groove and to remind you that cooking can be easy and good for you! From the few ideas I give you, feel free to experiment. Hopefully, these will kick-start you back in the kitchen, a place where I find the best quality time takes place.

(Note: I cook by looking and tasting; these recipes are so simple you should feel free to make them according to what tastes good to you.)

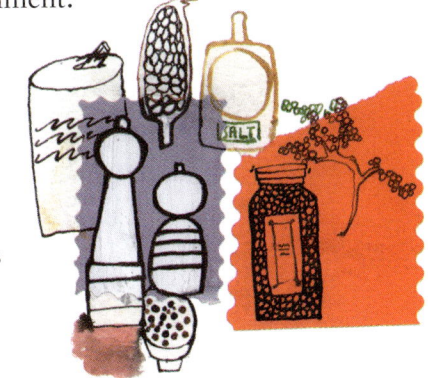

Breakfast

Muesli

One of the things the kids and I both love is Muesli and making our own together. Start with hazelnuts or almonds, raisins, and any other dried fruit you like—we like bananas and apricots but add whatever looks good. Mix in a bowl. (You may want to chop the ingredients a bit first.) Then add dried oatmeal (measure it out per the instructions on the box depending on how many people you're serving), some honey, cinnamon, and yogurt or milk if you like. One trick is to make a huge batch of it without the honey and yogurt, because you can store it like a normal cereal. Then add the yogurt or milk for each serving.

Another way to prepare this which my kids love is to put the mixture—minus the milk or yogurt—in the oven on a cookie sheet with a little brown sugar sprinkled on top. Cook for a few minutes at 450°F, and then serve. You can also use the extras as a snack for the kids in the afternoon! The nice thing about this recipe is that you're avoiding all the sugary cereal that supermarkets sell.

Marinades and Dressings

Often, I'll simply dress my salad with olive oil, balsamic vinegar, salt, and pepper. But here are a couple of dressings (one with almost no calories, the others with only a smidgen more, amazingly enough!) that are also great ways to marinate your chicken, fish, or meat before you grill it.

Soy Sauce and Ginger Dressing

Mix soy sauce and balsamic vinegar in a dish. Add pepper to taste; squeeze in a bit of lemon. Then grate or chop a teaspoon of ginger into the sauce. Adjust the ingredients to your taste. If you have a chance to let it sit for about 20 minutes, the ginger's flavor will seep into the liquid, but it's still filled with flavor if you use it immediately. As I said, this is great on vegetables, but you can also cook your chicken or fish in it.

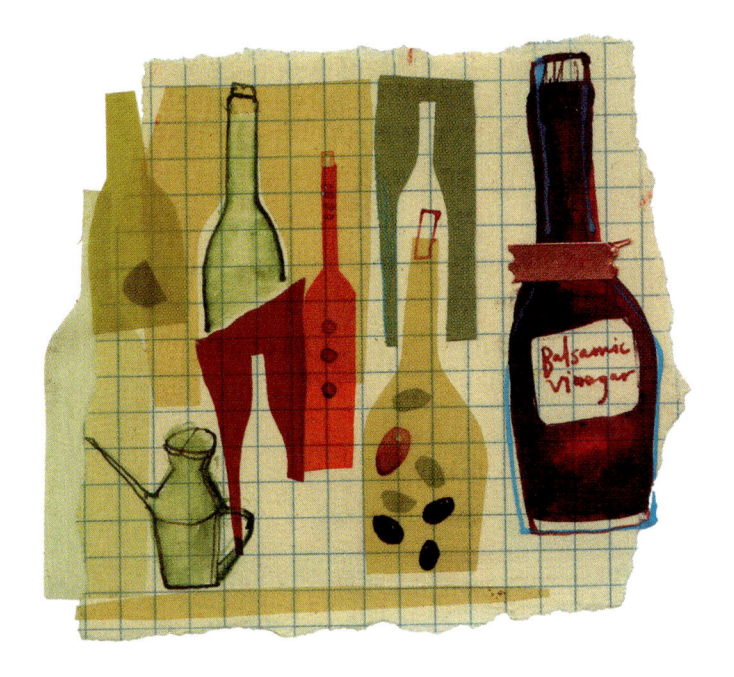

Mustard Vinaigrette

Again, this is a tasty way to spice up a salad or your meat. With a fork, whisk a teaspoon of olive oil and a few teaspoons of vinegar into a couple teaspoons mustard (Dijon packs the most taste, I think). Don't feel like you have to measure—you can add more where you need to according to your taste. Squeeze in a bit of lemon, and add salt and pepper to taste. While the Soy Sauce and Ginger Dressing will marinate your meats, this is a perfect sauce to apply directly on top of your chicken or fish before you put it under the broiler.

Soups

There's nothing like a warm bowl of soup to make you feel cared for and content. It also smells great when it's cooking, with not that much effort.

Chicken Soup

This is a guaranteed hit with kids and grown-ups. Buy a whole chicken; after washing carefully and patting dry with paper towels, put in a large soup pot. Add celery, peeled carrots, potatoes, a clove of peeled garlic, and a little bit of salt and pepper and cover with water. Cook for 40 minutes to 1 hour—you'll know when it's ready because the meat will be coming off the bone. Remove the chicken skin, add a little parsley, and you're good to go.

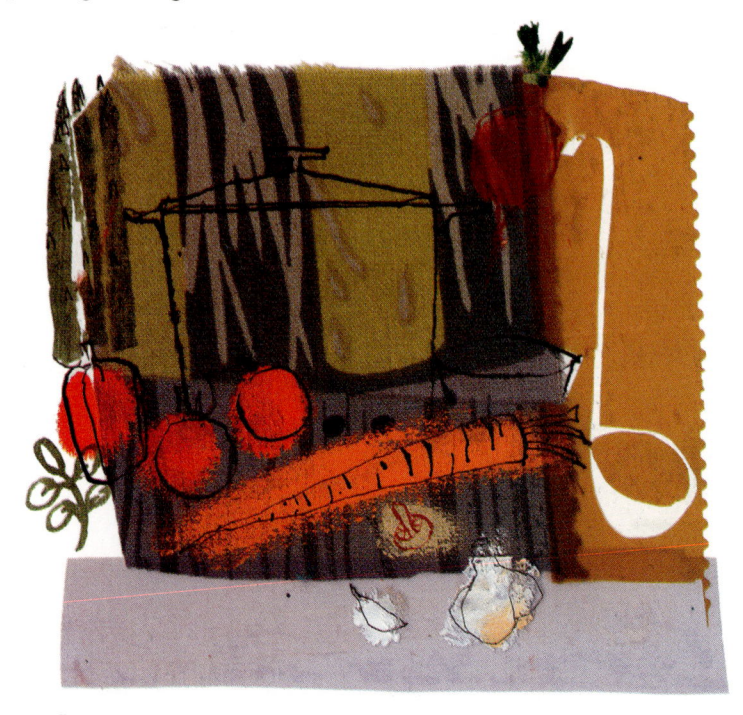

Chicken Noodle Soup

This variation for Chicken Soup is great for the whole family, especially when winter hits and everyone is threatening to catch a cold. The noodles make it fun for kids so they don't feel like they're getting something good for them. And it's incredibly fast, which is clearly one of our top priorities!

Simply boil some chicken breasts—however many will feed your clan—in a soup pot of water. When the chicken is almost cooked through—it should get tender and fall apart a bit—throw in a chopped clove of garlic, a couple teaspoons of ginger, chopped celery, and carrots. Continue to cook for about another 10 minutes or until the chicken is cooked through and the vegetables, ginger, and garlic have made a tangy broth. Then add angel hair pasta and cook for 2 minutes until it's done; turn off the heat and add about half a cup of cilantro if you can find it. If not, parsley will do. Season as you like it, and serve!

Super Fast, Super Easy Vegetable Soup

The great thing about this recipe isn't just that it's easy, it's that you can take the vegetables, which are cut into large pieces, out of the broth and give them to your infant to eat at his or her highchair. They'll be deliciously flavored and healthy too!

You will need some potatoes, zucchini, leeks, and an onion (feel free to add carrots or celery, if that sounds appealing, or anything else that looks good). In a heavy stockpot, sauté the vegetables in a little bit of olive oil just long enough to make sure they're all coated with the olive oil and slightly cooked—maybe 10 minutes. Add a bit of water if you sense the vegetables are getting burned. Then, fill the pot with water and stir occasionally. Once the water gets hot enough, stir in vegetable or chicken bouillon cubes (how many depends on how many cups of soup you're making), and cook for anywhere from 20 minutes to a couple of hours, depending on how much time you have. This soup is not only easy and tasty but also extremely low in calories, since it's just fresh vegetables. It's equally good in the winter when vegetables aren't as high-quality as in the summer.

Butternut Squash Soup

One of my favorite soups to serve is a butternut squash puree, which is rich and creamy without actually containing anything high in fat. It's also, like everything else here, incredibly easy to make, but looks and tastes comforting to the children and elegant to the adults.

Buy one large butternut squash. Preheat the oven to 400°F, and prick the squash with a fork in different places so it doesn't expand and blow up in the oven (a serious mess!). Put the squash directly on the rack, turning occasionally until the skin softens and begins to blister—about 15 minutes.

Skin and core the squash, cutting it into small chunks. Place the pieces in a sauté pan on top of the stove with enough chicken broth to cover the pieces (using bouillon cubes is fine). Add salt and pepper—a little bit of curry powder is a nice addition, as well—and let cook until the squash is soft. Run the soup through the blender and serve with a dollop of nonfat yogurt on top. This soup freezes beautifully, so make extra if you can!

Gazpacho

This is one of nature's greatest gifts in the summer months when tomatoes are ripe. If you make the gazpacho a bit thicker, it doubles as a lovely salsa to serve with rice or over chicken and fish. It's also as simple as turning your blender on!

There are a lot of different ways to make gazpacho, but I think the best is the simplest, because the flavors of the tomatoes really come through. (It's occasionally recommended that you add tomato juice, but my feeling is that if the tomatoes aren't perfectly ripe and juicy on their own, it's not worth making this soup in any case.) Cut up the tomatoes into quarters and put in the blender; add some chopped onion, pieces of cilantro, a cut up green pepper, salt, pepper, and the juice of a lemon. I occasionally add a dash of balsamic vinaigrette, which gives the tomatoes a nice flavor. Puree until the consistency is what you want—you don't want to blend it too much or it will turn out a bit mushy; I like to be able to still taste the chunks of the tomatoes and peppers, but adjust the consistency and seasoning as you go.

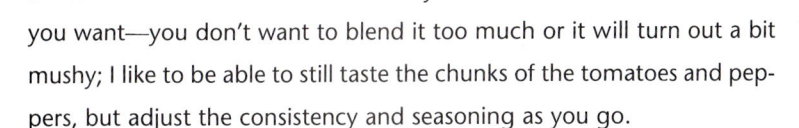

White Bean Soup

Soak a bag of white beans overnight in water, per the package's instructions. Then, when you're ready, heat in a large pot chicken stock; when the stock is heated, add the beans, a teaspoon of olive oil, a clove or two of crushed garlic, and one finely chopped carrot. Let the soup cook at a low boil for about 40 minutes. If you like, you can add a tasty sausage toward the end. Taste the beans to make sure they're cooked through and season with salt and pepper. This is a really big winner with my kids, and my husband and I love it too!

Cream of Cauliflower Soup

Take a whole cauliflower and chop it into bite-sized pieces. Boil the cauliflower in chicken stock until it's cooked through, about 20 minutes, and then add a chopped garlic clove and a splash of milk. Then place the mixture in the blender until it has a creamy consistency, add some salt and pepper, and you're done!

Main Courses
Chicken

Chicken may sound boring, but believe me, it can be your best friend in the kitchen when you've got only a little time. It's easy to get your hands on, it's ridiculously simple to flavor, and it'll cook up fast. Here are some of my favorite recipes that get me out of the kitchen in half an hour flat—including cooking time—but make me look like quite the fancy chef.

With all of these recipes, remember to add an extra chicken breast so you can snack on it the following day.

Poached Chicken Breasts

Poaching chicken meat is great because the chicken gets so tender, it's especially easy for a child who's not up to heavy-duty chewing! It's also a breeze, since it's done on your stove, and it is very low fat. Season your chicken breasts with a bit of olive oil (just for flavor), salt, pepper, and some chopped garlic. In a sauté pan, cook a garlic clove in just a dab of butter, adding a cup or two of chicken broth before the garlic burns. (The amount will depend on how many chicken breasts you're cooking; allow the breasts to sit in the broth while not being covered by it.) Bring the broth to a slow boil before adding the chicken; turn the heat down a bit and cover the pan. Allow the chicken breasts to cook for about 10 minutes or until the meat is cooked through.

Roasted Chicken

There are few things more beloved by all ages than a simple roasted chicken, but it's hard to find the time to season and grill an entire bird. One trick to cut down on cooking time but still get the great flavor is to buy chicken parts with the skin still on. Rub the chicken parts with a little bit of butter or olive oil, add some rosemary or thyme, salt, and pepper, and place at the top of a roasting pan. Underneath, add just enough chicken broth to cover the bottom of the pan, and place into that celery, carrots, leeks—whatever vegetables you like that will cook at the same time as the chicken. Cook at around 400°F until the meat is cooked through. I start checking at around 20 minutes, but it can take longer if the meat is in larger pieces. The meat and vegetables will have the taste you crave, and you'll cut down your cooking time by about an hour compared to if you were serving a whole chicken. And you don't have to carve it when it's time to eat!

Chicken and Vegetable Skewers

These are great for kids' parties. They are also great for getting your children into the kitchen to help, because it's fun for them to put the food on the skewers. First, buy the skewers; most vegetable stores will carry them. Cut chicken breasts into bite-size pieces and squeeze a bit of lemon on them. When I'm feeling inspired, I sometimes marinate the chicken in a little honey, too. Cut up a green pepper and whatever other vegetables you like—my children love zucchini and yellow squash and asparagus (weird, I know). I avoid onion because the kids don't like it. Place the food in alternating patterns on the skewer and cook in a roasting pan or on a cookie sheet at 450°F for 20 minutes or until the chicken is cooked through.

Indian Chicken

Skip ordering out—this is a wonderfully flavorful way to cook chicken in minutes flat. First, make the marinade—you have all the ingredients already: Into a cup of plain yogurt, add a dash of yellow mustard, paprika, and cumin; squeeze in a bit of lemon and season with salt and pepper.

Place your washed and dried chicken breasts into the marinade; if you have time to let the chicken sit in the marinade for an hour or so, all the better, but you can also use it immediately. Pour more of the marinade on top of the chicken so it's covering it. Put the chicken into the broiler and cook for about 20 minutes (test for doneness by cutting open the largest piece of chicken; a clear liquid should come out). The yogurt will get browned on top and will have coated the chicken so the chicken will be incredibly moist inside.

Chicken Breasts with Soy Sauce Marinade

Remember that marinade I mentioned earlier? Put some in the bottom of a pan and place your chicken breasts on top of it. Throw the chicken in the broiler for about 20 minutes or until it's cooked; occasionally spoon the marinade over the chicken while it's cooking. Done!

Lime and Ginger Chicken

This dish is easy and tasty, and it looks gorgeous. Marinate chicken breasts in lime juice, balsamic vinegar, and a little fresh ginger. Add salt and pepper and throw it in a Ziploc bag to marinate for the day if you can (an hour will do it, but the chicken will get more tender if you can leave it a few hours). Then put the chicken in a sauté pan with olive oil and cook on medium heat (check to see that it's done the way you like; I prefer to cook only until it's a little pink inside and then let it finish cooking in the hot pan off the heat). Start checking after 5 to 7 minutes. Let the chicken sit for a bit, then cut into pieces and garnish the chicken with the extra lime.

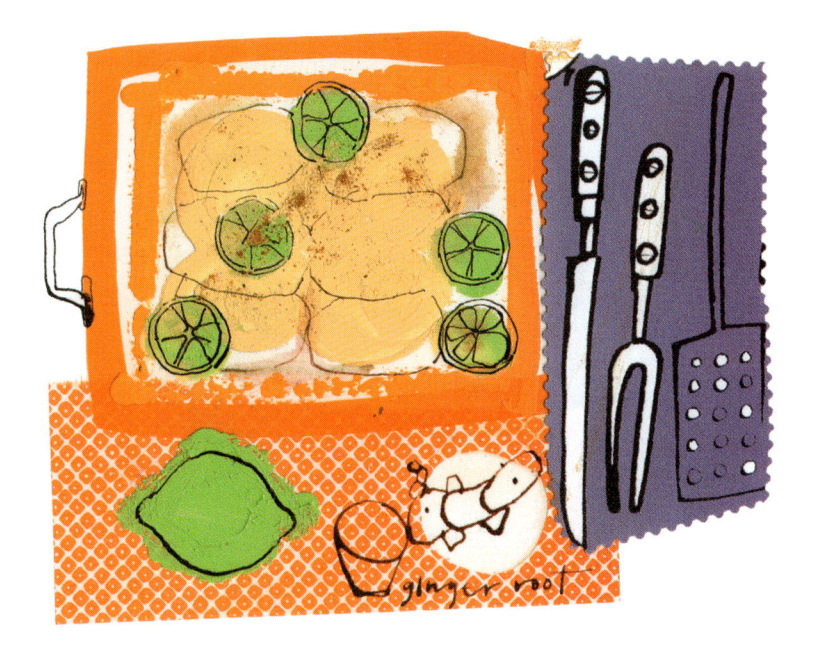

Julia loves this with rice; when I'm not eating too many carbohydrates, I'll eat it with an arugula salad.

Turkey

Turkey Hamburgers

This is a great way to avoid red meat when you feel like you've eaten too much of it, without having your family feel like they're getting healthfooded to death. Take some ground turkey and add in a little salt and pepper, finely chopped onion, and a pepper—they add a fun crunch. Form into patties and put in the broiler until cooked through, using a fork to test. Serve with toasted bread (or buns, if you really want to fool them!). This dish is low fat, as easy and as fast as a meal comes, and the kids love it if you put out the usual ketchup and pickles they're used to! (I also sometimes use fresh tuna to make tuna burgers; simply combine the fish with the vegetables and seasoning in the blender, and then form the patties.)

Turkey Meatloaf

This meal is a wonderful thing to serve when winter sets in and you're longing for comfort food.

Preheat the oven to 350°F. Buy 1 pound of ground turkey meat—the low-fat is perfect; nonfat is too dry. Using your hands, combine the turkey with chopped garlic, salt, pepper, one egg, and any vegetables that you want to get rid of in the refrigerator, which you've blended in the cuisinart so they're finely chopped (if they're too large, it interferes with the texture of the meat). Mushrooms, carrots, celery, onions—anything you've got in the vegetable cooler is great! Mold into a loaf and place in a lightly greased bread pan. On top, place a thin layer of chili sauce (Heinz is good). Cook at 350°F for approximately 35 minutes, checking occasionally to make sure the loaf doesn't get too dry. Let the turkey loaf sit for 15 minutes so the juices don't run out all over the plate when you serve it.

Julia and Hannah's Grandmother's Turkey

This isn't a calorie saver, but I love having it for the holidays, when you just have to throw your weight watching to the side.

When I met Olaf, his mother had passed away, but I had heard all these stories about her because she was a famous politician in Norway and France for working with asylum seekers. Our first Christmas together, Olaf wanted me to make his mother's turkey recipe, so I did a dry run a few days before and was stunned at how delicious and easy it was. My children, who never knew their grandmother, know this is her turkey and think of her every time I serve it.

Buy a turkey at the grocery store or from your local butcher. For the stuffing, put in a bowl a pound of ground beef, a cup of chestnut puree, a lot of garlic (about five cloves, finely chopped), a splash of cognac if you have it, salt, and pepper. Mix all these things together. The family insists that the turkey has to be stuffed the night before, but I don't do it because of the risk of salmonella. Stuff the turkey, and then take a half a package of bacon slices and stuff it under the skin as much as you're able. I add a yellow onion into the turkey's cavity to block the stuffing from coming out. Cook it in a roasting pan in the oven for the appropriate amount of time—ask at the meat counter for how long is right for the weight of your bird—occasionally basting the turkey with the juices. I promise you'll have the best turkey of your life! Now, if you want to do this the traditional way, you serve it with potato chips instead of mashed potatoes, and green peas. I also sauté whole chestnuts with brown sugar and honey in a pan and brown them. I admit it's high in caloric intake, but it's worth every bite!

Fish

In Sweden and Norway, where I come from, fish is a huge part of our cuisine, and I was surprised when I came to the United States to find how much people don't like it. But I'm pretty sure that's because until recently, it was hard to get fresh fish in the grocery store; it came frozen, when it had lost it's flavor and tasted really fishy.

Most grocery stores now sell fresh fish fillets, and if you haven't taken advantage of it before, now is a perfect time because fish is low in fat and calories and so good for you. Plus, it's one of the easiest things to prepare.

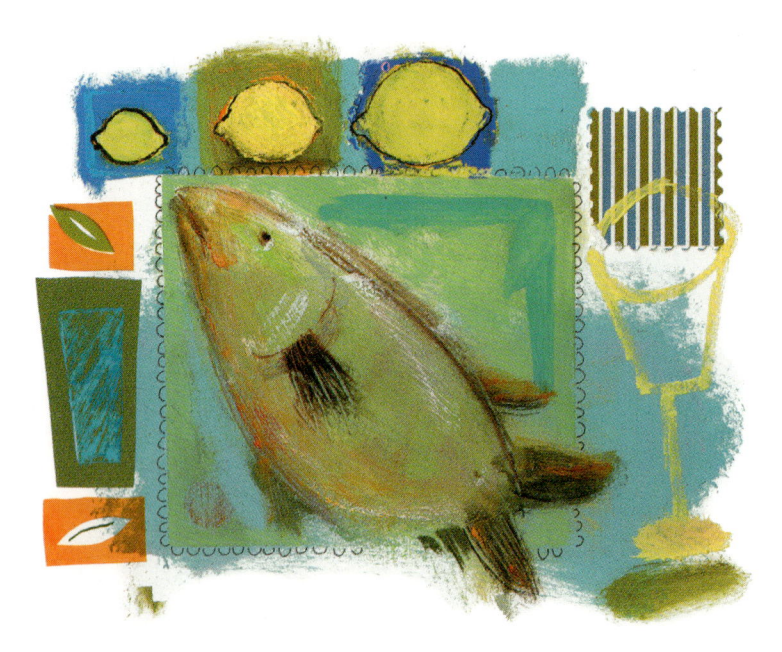

Fillet of Sole

Here's a perfect example of a way to cook for you, your toddler, and your husband that takes minutes but makes everyone happy! For me, I'll take a fillet of sole and put on it lemon juice, a little olive oil, salt, and pepper and put it under the broiler for 10 minutes. (In terms of grilling or broiling fish this way, it works equally well with snapper, salmon, or anything else that appeals to you.)

For my daughter, I'll dip the fish in bread crumbs and cook it in a bit of butter on top of the stove. It's hard to believe it's that easy, right? You can do it in your sleep (which you may be doing, anyway, at this point!) and still serve up a meal everyone loves. If you use chicken instead of sole, you have a recipe for delicious chicken nuggets.

Salmon in Foil

Again, this recipe is extremely easy, and almost any fish can be used. But the reason it's one of my favorites is that it's so easy to clean up—just throw out the foil and you're done! Buy a fillet of salmon; cut up some fresh dill to put on top and add a little salt and pepper. Then add thin slices of lemon (include the rind). Place the fillet in a piece of aluminum foil and wrap it up like a present. Throw it in the oven at 450°F for about 10 minutes, and that's that!

Tuna in a Soy Sauce Marinade

This is easy but also very elegant, so it's a good trick to have in your hat if you need to pull together a nice dinner quickly. In a broiling pan, combine soy sauce (you can opt for the low-sodium brand, if you prefer), lemon juice, a little grated ginger if you have some on hand, a chopped garlic clove, and salt and pepper. Wash the tuna steaks thoroughly and pat them dry before placing them down in the pan. Put in the refrigerator to marinate—it's best if you have an hour, but not necessary if you're rushed for time; the flavor will still be delicious—rotating the tuna so both sides absorb the marinade. Put under the broiler and cook—depending on how rare you like your tuna and how thick the slices are, this could be 3 minutes or 8 minutes (again, check with a fork as it cooks). When it's cooked to your liking, simply drain whatever extra marinade there is. Try it with rice or couscous or potatoes. It's also delicious the next day for lunch.

Meat

Swedish Meatballs

OK, *this* I'm an expert in. This dish is high in protein and very satisfying. In a medium-size bowl, combine bread crumbs and a little milk; let the mixture sit for 5 minutes until the crumbs are a little soggy. Add lean ground beef and an egg and mix it up, adding a little soy sauce and pepper as you do. Make little meat patties and sauté in a pan. Then, when the meatballs are cooked through, take yours out; leave your child's in (and your husband's, if he didn't gain too much sympathy weight while you were pregnant), and add a little heavy cream to the sauce. Cook for a few more minutes and serve. This is really good with boiled potatoes and carrots cooked with a little dill. To complete the meal you might also add a cucumber salad tossed with a little white wine vinegar, a dash of sugar, lemon, and dill.

Thai Meatballs

To make Thai meatballs, chop fresh cilantro (also called coriander) and put it in a bowl; add a little soy sauce, chopped ginger, and garlic, along with the bread crumbs soaked in milk (see Swedish Meatballs). Throw in lean ground beef, mix it up, and cook as described above. If you feel like getting fancy, chop some unsalted peanuts or cashews and add a sprinkle of that to the mix.

It's nice to add some peanuts to a salad to accompany the Thai meatballs; a mango and onion salad, if your kids don't think that's too weird, is also a great accompaniment.

Both Swedish and Thai meatballs are great snacks to have around. Throw them on some bread with lettuce and they make great lunches the next day for you and your kids.

Lamb Stew

I've never met a kid who didn't like this, and again, it's a high-protein, low-fat dish for you. Buy lamb meat on the bone, which will add a great flavor to the broth. Tell your butcher it's for a stew, and ask him to cut the meat into pieces but keep the bone.

Chop a large yellow onion and three carrots and put in a stew pot along with the meat and the bone; add just enough water to cover the meat, and flavor with salt and pepper. Cover and cook on medium heat for at least 2 hours. Keep an eye on it in case you need to add a little more water, but the more you cook it, the more tender it will be. The lamb will take on the consistency of a very soft vegetable; if you mash a potato and add a little broth, your kids will be in heaven.

Roasted Leg of Lamb

This is such a hearty meal, and again, one you won't have to give much thought to at all. Ask the butcher for a leg of lamb—make sure it's not too big to fit in your oven, a mistake I've made! Preheat the oven to 450°F, and season the leg with salt and pepper. Adding a little rosemary can be nice, if you like. Place the lamb in a roasting pan (vegetables below, like with the roasted chicken, if you like; adding potatoes to the mix here can be really good and easy). Cook at 450°F for 20 minutes, then reduce the temperature to 350°F. Cook for another hour, or until the lamb is done to your liking. Fancy cooks use meat thermometers, but it's just as simple to put a knife and fork into the thickest piece of meat to check on it.

Veal Cutlets

This is incredibly fast, low in calories and fat, and everyone in the family will be delighted. Preheat the oven to 350°F. Take veal cutlets pounded by your butcher or pound them yourself (put them between two pieces of wax paper and whack them with a soup can or a rolling pin until they're as thin as can be). Put them in a nonstick baking pan and drizzle olive oil, salt, and pepper on both sides of the veal. Add the juice of one lemon, sprinkle with capers, some olives if you like, and a whole garlic clove. Put them in the oven; after 5 minutes, flip the cutlets (they're thin, so they cook fast), and cook for another 5 minutes until they're browned. Perfect with roasted vegetables!

Pork Chops

All kids love pork chops, and they're not that fatty if you get lean cuts. Simply preheat the oven to 350°F. Salt and pepper both sides of the pork chops and cover with rosemary twigs. Bake for 10 minutes on each side (or ask your butcher the exact baking time, since it can vary a bit, depending on the size of the meat) until browned. Potatoes go great with this dish.

Pizza

Mini Pizzas

I got this recipe for mini pizzas from Julia's godfather. They are great for the kids' birthdays because they can be involved in making them, but we also love to just hang out on the weekends and do this as a family.

The secret is the dough. Take one packet of fresh yeast, a cup of water, and two cups of flour—you can add a little more flour or water if it's too wet or too dry while you mix it together—and half teaspoon of salt. Mix together with your hands until it's well incorporated: it should be soft but not gooey. (If it sticks to your hands too much, add a bit more flour.) Knead the dough into a ball and then drizzle olive oil on top so it's nice and moist. Leave the dough in the bowl with a cloth draped over the top and place it on top of your refrigerator where the mixture will be warm. Let stand for at least two hours. Then, it's on to the fun. Roll out the dough and add the toppings. From tomato sauces to cheeses to vegetables, it's all fair game. Roasted vegetables are wonderful on top. Making your own pizza is perfect because adults watching their weight can do cheeseless pizza, but the kids can have all the cheese they want! Preheat the oven to 450°F and cook the pizzas on a baking pan low in the oven for about 10 minutes.

(The dough freezes well so make extra for next time. You can also use this dough to wrap around little hotdogs for pigs in a blanket for the children—a sure hit!)

Side Dishes

Rice

I also really like rice, but I'm a terrible rice cooker, as I suppose every new mother is (who has the concentration to watch for the precise moment when it's done?). I ruined more pots than I can count by scorching them, until I finally invested in a rice steamer. Let me tell you, it's one of the great inventions of our century! Try brown rice when you can, since it packs more nutrients than white.

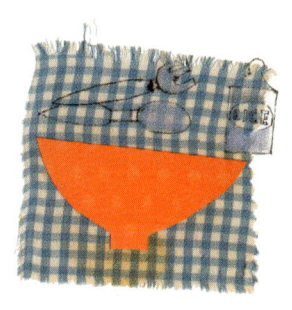

Steamed Vegetables

For me, vegetables are really the way to go—you just cut up the vegetables of your choice, steam them, and voilà! For the children, I add a little butter for taste.

Roasted Vegetables

Nothing is easier or more delicious as a side dish than roasted vegetables. Roast up a slew of vegetables and you can serve them for the next couple of days at room temperature. I like to get whatever is fresh in the market, but the nice thing about roasting vegetables is that the winter selection of produce—usually sad compared to summer's stock—cooks up beautifully.

The best vegetables for this include zucchini, squash, leeks, and mushrooms; any root vegetable works as well. Clean the vegetables and then slice. Put the slices in a bowl and toss with a bit of olive oil, sea salt if you have it (the larger-grained salt works nicely when you're roasting), and chopped garlic. Lay the vegetables down on a baking pan or a piece of tin foil and place in the broiler, or in the oven at around 450°F. Cook until the edges start to brown a bit. The squash will cook fairly quickly, while the root vegetables will take longer, usually about 10 minutes. Flip the vegetables occasionally so they cook thoroughly, and then serve. A dollop of goat cheese alongside the vegetables can add a lovely creamy texture to the richness of the roasted flavor.

The day after you make the vegetables, try this trick: boil some pasta and toss the vegetables in with it—you'll have a very tasty pasta primavera in about 8 minutes!

Vegetables Simmered in Chicken Broth

Start by making the broth. You can use vegetable or chicken bouillon cubes, whichever you prefer. Both add a wonderful flavor. The best vegetables for this tend to be leeks, which grow sweet and tender, carrots, and celery. Make enough vegetable or chicken broth to cover the vegetables in a pan and heat it up on the stove. Add the leeks (make sure to clean them thoroughly!), carrots, and celery, and cook in the broth until the carrots grow soft but not gummy. Drain the remaining liquid and serve!

Green Vegetable Casserole

You can use anything for this baked dish from asparagus to green swiss chard (if you use the swiss chard be sure to remove the leaves—you want only the stalks). Preheat the oven to 400°F. Lay the vegetables in a lightly buttered baking dish, so they're lying flat next to one another. Sprinkle with a little parmesan cheese. The great thing about good, sharp parmesan is a little goes a long way, so don't worry about the calories. Continue to layer the vegetables until you're out. Bake until the cheese browns and the vegetables are cooked—about 15 minutes. Your children won't even notice they're eating greens the dish is so good!

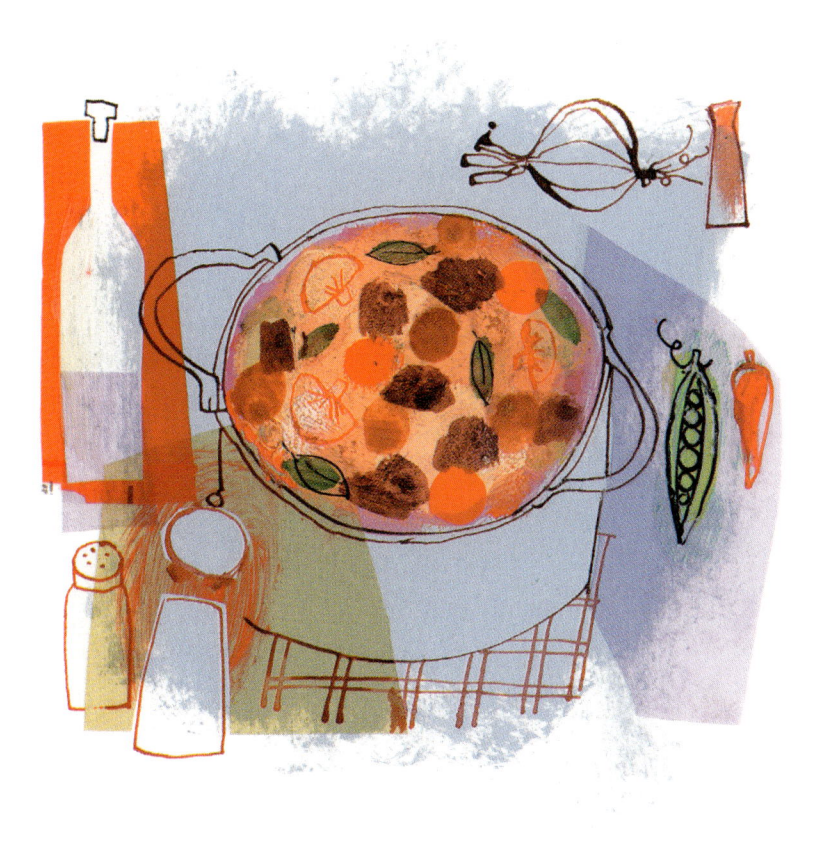

Potatoes

I also eat a lot of potatoes. Here's a delicious alternative to french fries: instead of frying them in vegetable oil, cut up the potatoes and put them in a baking dish. Drizzle olive oil, salt, and pepper over them, and bake them for 45 minutes or so (keep an eye on them, since cooking time will depend on how thick they're cut). They'll be as crispy and tasty as french fries, promise! And the leftovers make great midnight snacks. You can substitute sweet potatoes for a nice change and to gain lots of great vitamins.

Potatoes with Pesto

This recipe is great because you get the flavor of a wonderful pasta without the empty carbohydrates (I also leave out the pine nuts for lower calories when I'm counting). Take a handful of basil and one or two cloves of chopped garlic and place in a blender. Then, as it chops, slowly add olive oil until the mixture has the consistency of a paste. Add salt and pepper. Set aside. Now boil the potatoes (the little red ones are the most flavorful, I think). I scrub them but leave the skin on for the extra protein. Drain the water out of the potatoes and mix the pesto throughout—but use it sparingly because it's strong! For the children, I usually add a little freshly grated parmesan on top. The pesto can also double as a really flavorful marinade on chicken breasts.

Swedish Pancakes

We eat this dish as a main course with a salad or a soup first, although it's more like a dessert in North America. In Sweden, it's traditional to eat these on Thursday evenings. Take two eggs, ½ cup flour, ¼ cup milk, and a dash of salt and sugar. Mix together with a whisk. Then, ladle out one at a time and place in a sauté pan with a little bit of butter—it's similar to cooking pancakes, but remember that Swedish pancakes are much thinner, more like French crepes (and much better, if you ask me!). Flip the pancake over when you see little bubbles, until both sides are golden. Then add berries, jam, or a little sugar and lemon. A fun thing for the children is to leave the toppings on the table so that they can add their own topping.

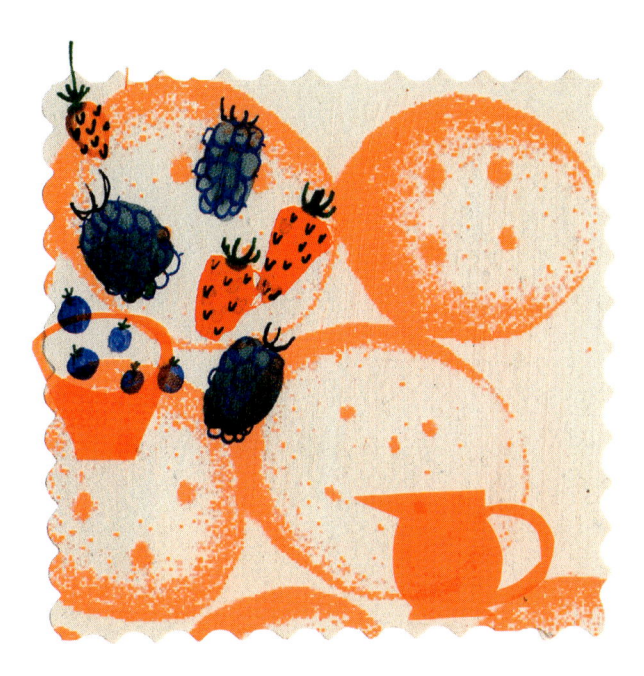

Desserts

It's totally possible to serve desserts your whole family will love that won't have you running an extra mile at the gym tomorrow.

Baked Apples

A perfect example of a dessert that feels decadent but isn't is baked apples. Peel and core the apples; into the core add raisins, cinnamon, a little lemon juice, and a drizzle of honey. Put under the broiler until they become mushy and sweet. For your kids, if they'd like, serve with a dollop of ice cream.

Grilled Bananas

Another easy sweet dessert is grilled bananas: Cut the bananas in half, add a little brown sugar, and put under the broiler until the brown sugar melts, about 5 minutes.

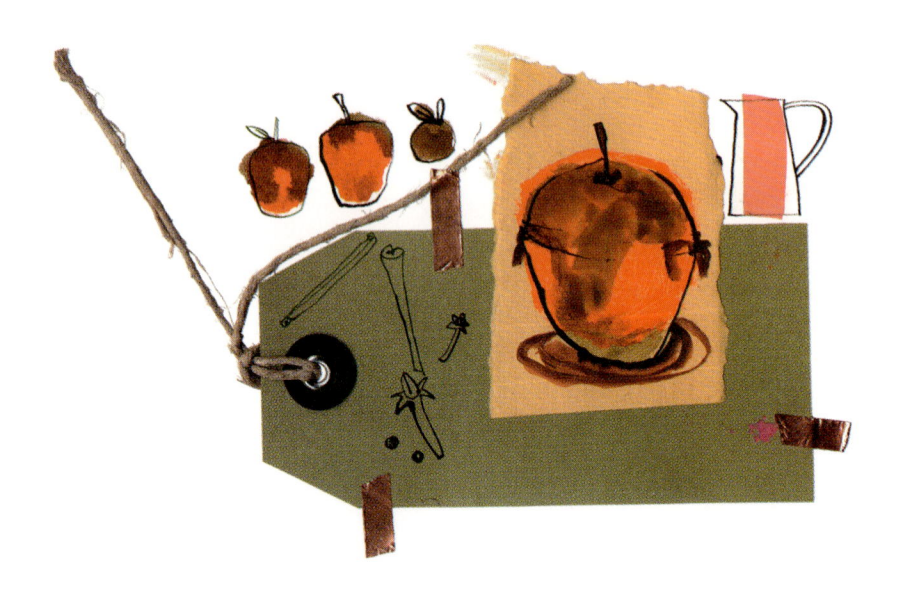

Fruit Salad

Here's a fruit salad that your kids will love. Peel and slice oranges; put the slices in a bowl with nuts and raisins and mix. Serve with fat-free sour cream and honey on the side.

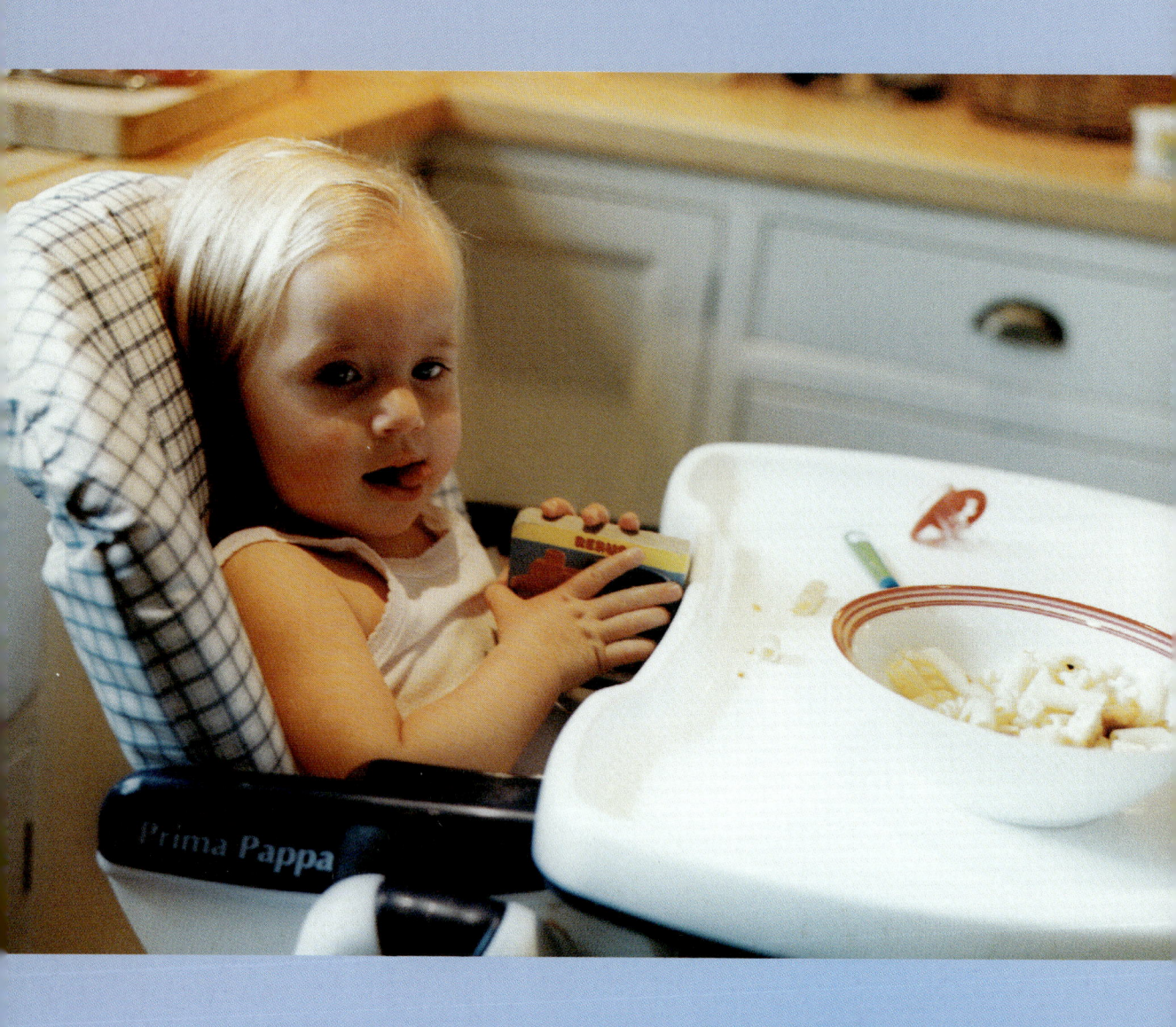

17

Cooking Your Own Baby Food

For me, making my own baby food is less expensive, and it's better for my kids. Plus I can freeze it, make extra, and do it at the same time I'm cooking my own meals. I promise, this doesn't have to be complicated, and it's a great way to start your kids on a life of enjoying delicious food. It's never too early to develop taste buds.

When your children are very small, of course, they need baby food, which is so simple to make. First, invest in a blender. Then there's very little you're eating that you can't make wonderful for your child too. At first, it's best not to mix too many ingredients together. Keep it simple, so your child is having one taste at a time, and you can be sure he or she isn't having an allergic reaction to something.

If the food is solid, add a little chicken bouillon or vegetable bouillon when you blend it to make the consistency easier for your child to swallow. Cook up an apple, or throw a pear and a banana in a blender, and you'll have a baby smoothie. Not only will your baby love the food, but you'll feel extremely wholesome having done it yourself! (Your friends will also be impressed, and there's no reason to tell them it didn't take more than thirty seconds.)

A great place to start is with sweet potatoes. Because they're so sweet, babies love them, and they're very high in vitamins and protein. Here's how easy it is: just throw a sweet potato in boiling water until a knife can go through it (to make it go faster, you can chop the potato into pieces). This works well for carrots, potatoes, and asparagus (stay away from broccoli because it can cause gas). Put the vegetable in a blender, along with a little bit of the water that it cooked in, and a smidgen of butter if you like, and blend until smooth. That's it, your done.

After a week or two you can start playing around, adding vegetables so you make a kind of medley. As the child gets older and more used to things, around eight months, start adding things like a piece of chicken, which you'll chop up into tiny pieces and boil along with the vegetables, or a small piece of the lamb that's left over from the lamb stew. After a year, I begin to add fish to my child's diet.

By making your own baby food, your whole family can enjoy the food that you prepare from the very beginning, even if one of you is a baby and another one of you is watching your weight. This is one more way food can bring the family together.

Appendix

And Away We Go! Traveling with Your Children

As my husband says, traveling with children is like being a roadie for the Rolling Stones—you're constantly unloading and loading boxes and suitcases! While I still haven't figured out how to get that great Rolling Stones concert at the end of our trips, I have traveled quite a bit with my children, especially since I bring them on location when I have to work. I wouldn't say it's ever a breeze, but I have learned some tips that work for us.

Travel at Night

My mother lives about three hours away from us, and early on my husband and I learned that the best trick was to drive at night. It gave us a peaceful trip, and it didn't disrupt the children's schedules, which, as you know, can take a lot longer to right again than the time of the entire trip!

If you must travel during the day, allow plenty of time and plan to stop for older babies and children to play. This can be very tricky if your child is crawling—not many places along the road tend to be clean enough for crawlers, so plan as best you can.

When we have to fly we take evening flights if we can because then the children are naturally sleepy. The one thing I would say about this is do whatever you have to to keep them awake during the time right before leaving the house and on the way to the airport. Otherwise, they won't sleep on the plane. I play games with them in the car, sing, or keep up as lively a conversation as I can with them until we're safely at the airport.

Always Plan Ahead

One way to avoid a sure drama is to make sure that you have booked your seats ahead of time; there's nothing worse than getting to the airport with two restless kids and having to do battle with the airlines. I take it to an even further extreme and order special meals twenty-four hours ahead of time, just to make sure our meals will be accounted for. Also, make sure to confirm the flight time before you leave the house. While it wasn't a big deal when you were flying solo to wait a couple extra hours in the airport, doing so unecessarily with children can make a wreck of you before you even get on the flight.

What to Bring on the Plane

Several items will prove useful on the plane and directly before and after the flight. Definitely plan to bring:

- The car seat. Bringing a car seat on the plane is bulky and it does cost more for your child to have his or her own seat, but it really helps. Most children are used to sitting still for at least some length of time in their own car seat, so the trip is more bearable than if you are juggling your little one in your lap or in a seatbelt that is too easily removed.

- The stroller. You can't bring this onto the plane as you can a car seat, but you can wheel it right up to the door of the plane and check it there. Most airlines will allow you to do this and will have it waiting for you as soon as you get off the plane at your destination. You will find this to be much easier than checking the stroller with your regular luggage because you won't have to carry children and carry-ons from the counter to the gate and onto the plane.

- Something for your child to chew or suck on. For young babies, have a bottle ready at take-off and landing to help their ears adjust to the change in pressure. Gum always works for children old enough to know not to swallow it.

Packing

While I try to pack as little as possible, there are some crucial tricks.

- If you can, pack a different suitcase for each of you, even if they're tiny. Then label them with your children's names. If you feel uncomfortable with strangers seeing the names use a special symbol so that you know whose is whose. While separate bags can be a little more unwieldy, it's worth it to know exactly which bag you need without having to pack and repack several times each day.
- The most important bag you pack is going to be your carry-on, since that's what you'll be left with should the airlines lose your luggage! One thing I've learned is that your carry-on bag should always be a backpack, because then your hands are free to wrangle children and strollers. The things you must have in the backpack are:

1. Enough diapers and wipes for two days
2. Toys for little babies and crayons, paper, and books for children old enough to color. To help them look forward to trips, I usually go with them to pick out new things, so they get excited about getting onto the plane and playing with them. I also let the girls each pick something they want to play with especially, so we avoid getting onto a plane and being stuck with things they aren't interested in.
3. A cosmetic bag with what the kids might need—but hopefully won't! That means a thermometer, baby acetaminophen or ibuprofen, and nose spray (children's noses can get stuffy on planes, which can lead to painful earaches).

4. Extra food. I always pack extra sandwiches just in case the plane doesn't have enough food or we get stuck sitting on the runway for a long time. Kids don't understand having to wait when they're hungry!
5. A small bag of candy. I don't usually like my children to have candy, but it can be very helpful when we're traveling to use sparingly as bribes! (Don't give them too much, or they will be bouncing out of their seats.) When there's chaos around and you have to get your toddler strapped into a seatbelt, there won't always be time to reason, especially if you're on a long trip and everyone is tired.
6. A change of clothing for each child. Invariably, someone spills or wets her pants or gets cold or hot. It's great to be able to change clothes when you're traveling if you need to, and if you don't, you're prepared to get through a day if your luggage doesn't arrive with you.

As for what to do with screaming children on airplanes, the only trick I've learned is that most passengers are far more compassionate than you might think—especially the ones with children. And I remind myself as often as need be to hang in, because I know things will get better!

Index

Abdominal muscles
    crunches for, 84–87
    stretches for, 48, 54, 95
Activity, choosing exercise, 43–45
Aerobic exercise program, 59, 60–62
Airplane. *See also* Traveling
    flying at night, 154
    traveling on, 155
Anxiety, 10, 12
Apples, baked, 148
Arm stretches, 55
Asparagus, 152

Baby
    exercising with your, 89–99
    impact on life, 3–7
    impact on marriage, 17–23
    squats with, 94
Baby food, cooking your own, 151–52
Baked apples, 148
Ball crunches, 86
Balsamic vinegar, 118, 123
Bananas, grilled, 148
Basil, 124, 125
Beans, white, soup, 131
Biceps curls, 82

Binge, 110
Body fat, 62
Body image, boosting your, 25–29
Bottle feeding, 33
Breakfast, 126
    muesli, 126
Breast-feeding, 27, 31–35, 104, 107
    hot line for, 33
    hunger attacks and, 103
    in public, 33
Breast pumps, 33
Broccoli, 152
Butternut squash soup, 130

Cardio work, 57–63, 65
Carrots, 152
Car seat, traveling with, 155
Casserole, green vegetable, 145
Cauliflower, cream of, soup, 131–32
Chair in squats, 70
Chicken, 107, 132–35, 152
    breasts with soy sauce marinade, 134
    Indian, 134
    lime and ginger, 134–35

noodle soup, 129
poached, breasts, 132
roasted, 133
soup, 128
strips, 107
and vegetable skewers, 133
vegetables simmered in, broth, 144
Children
care of, by father, 19–21
traveling with, 153–57
flying on airplane, 155
at night, 154
packing for, 156–57
planning in, 154–55
Chocolate, 107, 109–10
Compromise, 14
Cooking
for two and a half, 117–21
for whole family, 115
Cream of cauliflower soup, 131–32
Crunches, 84, 85
with baby, 92–93
ball, 86
lower-ab ball, 86, 87
reverse, 84, 85
Crying, handling, 10
Cumin, 124
Curry, 124

Depression, exercise in combating, 41
Desserts, 147
baked apples, 148
fruit salad, 149
grilled bananas, 148
Diamond pushups, 84
Diet, 25

Dumbbell press, 75, 79
one-armed, 82–83

Eating disorders, 119
Eggs, 118
Emotions, hormones and, 3–7
Engorgement, 31, 33
Exercise, 25
aerobic, 59, 60–62
with baby, 89–99
cardio work, 57–63, 65
choosing activity you like, 43–45
in combating depression, 41
Keigel, 22
motivation for, 39–41
personal trainer in, 40, 92
strength training and, 57, 65–87
stretching and, 47–49
Exercise ball
for ball crunches, 86
for lower-ab ball crunches, 86, 87
pushups on, 78
in squats, 71–72

Fat burning, 60
Father
child care by, 19–21
feeding of child by, 21
involvement of, in parenting, 7
Feeding, father's time for, 21
Fillet of sole, 136–37
Fish, 107, 137–39
fillet of sole, 138
salmon in foil, 138–39
tuna in a soy sauce marinade, 139

160   *Index*

Foods
    cooking baby, 151–52
    enjoying your, 99–101
    indulgences and, 109–13
    stocking healthy, 103–7
Fruits, 107, 124
Fruit salad, 149

Gazpacho, 130–31
Ginger, fresh, 124
Green vegetable casserole, 145
Grilled bananas, 148
Gum, 155

Hamstring stretch, 49–51
Hand weights
    in biceps curls, 82
    in doing plies, 73
    in dumbbell presses, 75, 79
    in lateral raise, 80, 81
    in lunges, 75
    in one-armed dumbbell press, 82–83
    in upright row, 81
Help, asking for, 12–13
Herbs de Provence, 124, 125
Hip stretches, 52
Hormones, 3–7
Husband. *See also* Father
    involvement, in parenting, 7

Indian chicken, 134
Indulgences, 109–13
Inner thigh stretches, 54
IQ tests, 31

Julia and Hannah's grandmother's turkey, 136–37

Keigel exercises, 22

Lactic buildup and cramping, 48
Lamb, 152
    roasted leg of, 141
    stew, 140–41
Lateral raise, 80, 81
Lemon, 124
Lime and ginger chicken, 133–34
Limitations, accepting your, 13
Lists, making, 14
Lower-ab ball crunches, 86, 87
Lower back and glute stretches, 53
Luggage, 152–53
Lunges, 74–75
    with baby, 94
    walking, 75

Main courses
    chicken, 132–35
        breasts with soy sauce marinade, 134
        Indian, 134
        lime and ginger, 134–35
        poached, breasts, 132
        roasted, 133
        and vegetable skewers, 133
    fish, 137–39
        fillet of sole, 138
        salmon in foil, 138–39
        tuna in a soy sauce marinade, 139
    meat, 139–42
        lamb stew, 140–41
        pork chops, 142
        roasted leg of lamb, 141

Swedish meatballs,
139–40
Thai meatballs, 140
veal cutlets, 141–42
turkey, 135–37
hamburgers, 135–36
Julia and Hannah's
grandmother's,
136–37
meatloaf, 136
Marinades and dressings, 126–27
mustard vinaigrette, 127
soy sauce and ginger dressing,
126–27
Marjoram, 125
Marriage
impact of baby on, 17–23
scheduling time for each other
in, 18–19
sex drive and, 21–23
Maximum heart rate, 60
Mayonnaise, 121
Meat, 139–42
lamb stew, 140–41
pork chops, 142
roasted leg of lamb, 141
Swedish meatballs, 139–40
Thai meatballs, 140
veal cutlets, 141
Mini pizza, 142–43
Mood swings in pregnancy, 4–5
Mother. *See also* Parenting
asking, for help, 9
need for time alone, 19–21
Motivation
for exercise, 39–41
role of personal trainer in, 40
tips for, 41

Muesli, 126
Mustard vinaigrette, 127

Night, traveling at, 150
Nuts, 104–5

Oatmeal, 118
Olive oil, 118, 123
One-armed dumbbell press,
82–83
One Rules, 18
Oregano, 125

Packing for traveling, 156–57
Pancakes, Swedish, 146–47
Paprika, 124
Parenting, 9–15. *See also* Father,
Mother
involvement of husband in, 7
Parsley, dried, 124
Partner in doing squats, 69
Peanut butter, 107
Personal trainer, 40, 92
strength training and, 65–87
Pizza, mini, 142–43
Planning, travel and, 154–55
Plies, 72–74
hand weights in doing, 73
Poached chicken breasts, 132
Pork chops, 142
Postpartum checkup, 60
Potatoes, 146, 152
with pesto, 146
salad, 121
Pregnancy, mood swings in,
4–5
Protein, 104

Pushups, 75, 76–78
    diamond, 84
    on exercise ball, 78

Raisins, 104–5
Red pepper flakes, 124
Reverse crunches, 84, 85
Rice, 143
Roasted chicken, 133
Roasted leg of lamb, 141
Roasted vegetables, 143–44
Rosemary, 124, 125
Running, 44–45

Salad, fruit, 149
Salmon in foil, 138–39
Sex drive, 21–23
Side dishes, 143–47
    green vegetable casserole, 145
    potatoes, 146
    potatoes with pesto, 146
    rice, 143
    roasted vegetables, 143–44
    steamed vegetables, 143
    Swedish pancakes, 146–47
    vegetables simmered in chicken broth, 144
Sleep, need for, 13
Snacks, 106–7
Soups, 128–32
    butternut squash, 130
    chicken, 128
    chicken noodle, 129
    cream of cauliflower, 131–32
    gazpacho, 130–31
    super fast, super easy vegetable, 129–30
    white bean, 131

Soy sauce, 123
Soy sauce and ginger dressing, 126–27
Soy sauce marinade
    chicken breasts with, 134
    tuna in, 139
Spices, 124–25
Spot reduction, 67
Squats
    with baby, 94
    chair in, 70
    exercise ball in, 71–72
    partner in, 69
Steamed vegetables, 141
Strength training, 57, 65–87
    ball crunches, 86
    biceps curls, 82
    crunches, 84, 85
    diamond pushups, 84
    dumbbell press, 75, 79
    intensity in, 67
    lateral raise, 80, 81
    lower-ab ball crunches, 86, 87
    lunges, 74–75
    muscle groups in, 67
    one-armed dumbbell press, 82–83
    philosophy to perfect workout, 67
    plies, 72–74
    pushups, 75, 76–78
    range of motion in, 67, 75
    repetitions in, 66
    reverse crunches, 84, 85
    sets in, 66
    squats, 68–72
    starting position for, 68

upright row, 81
wall sit, 72
Stretches, 47–49
   ab, 48, 54, 95
   arm, 55
   hamstrings, 49–51
   hip, 52
   inner thigh, 54
   lower back and glute, 53
   upper body and chest, 55
Stroller, traveling with 151
Super fast, super easy vegetable soup, 129–30
Swedish meatballs, 139–40
Swedish pancakes, 146–47
Sweet potatoes, 152

Thai meatballs, 140
Thyme, 125
Tomatoes, gazpacho, 130–31
Traveling. *See also* Airplane
   with children, 153–57
      need for car seat, 155
      need for stroller, 155
Tuna in a soy sauce marinade, 139
Turkey, 135–37
   hamburgers, 135–36

Julia and Hannah's grandmother's, 136–37
meatloaf, 136

Upper body and chest stretches, 55
Upright row, 81

Veal cutlets, 141–42
Vegetables, 107, 124
   chicken and, skewers, 133
   green, casserole, 145
   roasted, 143–44
   simmered in chicken broth, 144
   steamed, 143
   super fast, super easy, soup, 129–30
Virgin olive oil, 123

Walking, 44–45
Walking lunges, 75
Wall sit, 72
Weight gain and loss, 25–29
White bean soup, 131

Yellow mustard seeds, 124
Yogurt, 107, 121, 123